Healing, Miracles and the Bite of the Gray Dog

Majid Ali, M.D.

One of America's foremost spokespersons for preventive medicine and author of the Life Span Library of the Scientific Basis of Health.

* *The Canary and Chronic Fatigue*
* *Life, Healing and Thinking Ants*
* *The Cortical Monkey and Healing*
* *The Ghoraa and Limbic Exercise*
* *What Do Lions Know About Stress?*
* *RDA: Rats, Drugs and Assumptions*
* *The Butterfly and Life Span Nutrition*
* *Fibromyalgia: On the Moustache of A Mouse*
* *Lifespan, Health and the Flying Crickets*
* *Healing, Miracles and the Bite of the Gray Dog*
* *Cholesterol Cats, Chelation Mice and the Heart*
* *The Principles and Practice of Integrative Medicine*
* *The Battered Bowel Ecosystem-Waving Away A Wandering Wolf*
* *Do Fish Know Water?*

Healing, Miracles and the Bite of the Gray Dog

Majid Ali, M.D.

- President and Professor of Medicine,
  Capital University of Integrative Medicine, Washington, D.C.
- Associate Professor of Pathology
  College of Physicians and Surgeons of Columbia University,
  New York
- Visiting Professor, LHQG Hospital, Guanzhou, China
- President, the American Academy of Preventive Medicine
- Chief of Staff, Institute of Preventive Medicine,
  Denville, New Jersey and New York City
- Fellow, Royal College of Surgeons of England
- Diplomate, American Board of Anatomic Pathology
- Diplomate, American Board of Clinical Pathology
- Diplomate, American Board of Environmental Medicine
- Diplomate, American Board of Chelation Therapy

Healing, Miracles and the Bite of the Gray Dog
Copyright © Majid Ali, 1997

All Rights Reserved

Library of Congress Catalog Card Number
96-095233
ISBN 1-879131-11-X

Ali, Majid
Healing, Miracles and the Bite of the Gray Dog
Majid Ali--1st ed.
Includes bibliographical references and index.
1. Miracles
2. Health
3. Healing
4. Stress
5. Headache
6. Anxiety
7. Depression
8. Panic Reactions
9. Autoregulation
10. Spirituality

10 9 8 7 6 5 4 3 2 1

Published in the USA by
LIFE SPAN PRESS
95 East Main Street, Denville, New Jersey 07834
(201) 586-9191 (800) 633-6226

AN ESSENTIAL NOTE

I ask that readers do not expect me or any other staff member at the Institute to perform any miracle or to cure their specific health disorders. At the Institute, we do not perform miracles—we only witness them.

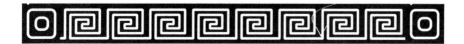

What Is A Miracle?

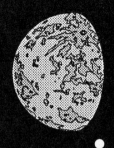

A miracle is but a glimpse of the infinite mystery of the one and only healer—the unknown and the unknowable. In this book I describe many such glimpses that the Institute staff and I were fortunate enough to have witnessed.

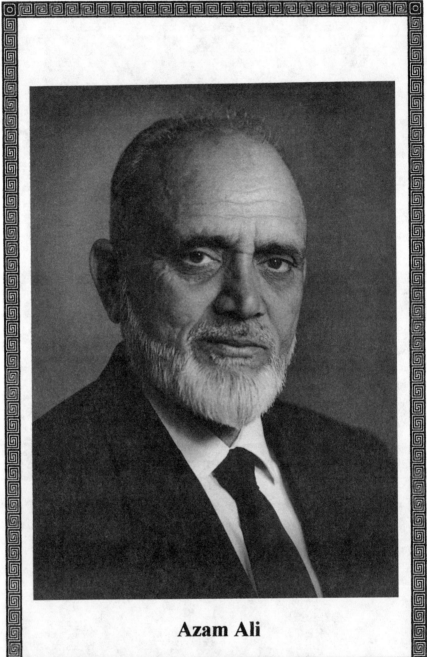

Azam Ali

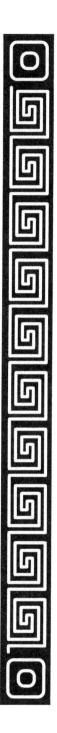

To my father,
Azam Ali,

Who urged me to pray for my patients when I was a young physician.

It took me nearly thirty years to recognize the profoundness of his advice.

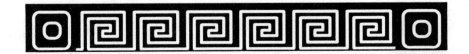

**To see a miracle,
you have to go past the mind.**

Miracles we witness multiply as our ability to witness grows.

Prayer
is the best antioxidant,

The scientific basis for this is simple:

Adrenaline is one of the most potent, if not the most potent, oxidant molecules in the human body. Prayer and meditation are the best ways to down-regulate adrenaline production.

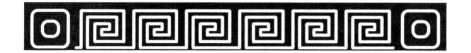

A Prayer

Lord, today may I simply be in your presence for a few moments.

Today I protest nothing.

Today I demand nothing.

Today may I simply be in your presence for a few moments.

The Canary and Chronic Fatigue

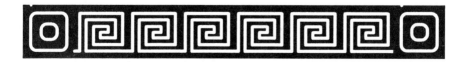

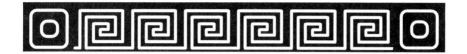

SCHUCKER

Give me the grace to treasure each breath.
Give me the grace to surrender each breath.

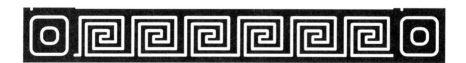

Progress in art and science requires two elements: a squint of the mind and selective deafness. The squint allows one to look at things others look at but see what no one else does; selective deafness saves one from the screams of reasonable men who cry 'foul.'

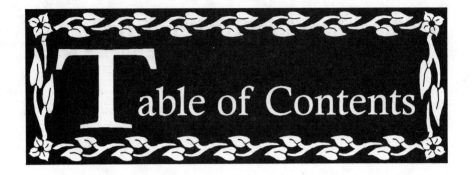

Table of Contents

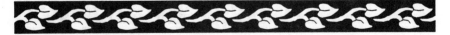

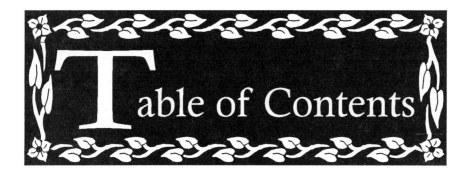

Table of Contents

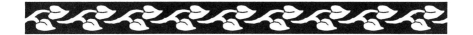

Healing, Miracles and the Bite of the Gray Dog

PREFACE

Of Dwarfs, Giants and Enlightenment

Miracles die in physician offices every day.

Miracles are usually defined as supernatural events that are outside the laws of nature. Since no one can claim to know *all* of the laws of nature, we must redefine miracles as supernatural events that are outside the *known* laws of nature. That, of course, raises another question: To whom are they known? In clinical medicine this becomes a critical issue.

Most physicians scoff at the plausibility of miracles in medicine. They accept drugs and surgical scalpels as the only legitimate agents for treating diseases. They promptly dismiss as chicanery any suggestion that healing occurred through any other medium. We physicians should recognize that when healing occurs as a supernatural event—supernatural to *us*—it should not be dismissed as an illusion, or worse, a deception perpetrated by a charlatan, simply because we fail to understand the mechanism of the healing phenomenon. We should also recognize that when we deny the possibility of miracles in medicine, our patients pay dearly for our narrowly focused and severely limited view of health, disease and healing.

When life begins, it begins to end. Life is a never ending cycle of injury-healing-injury continuum. I wrote those lines in my introduction to the companion volume, *What Do Lions Know About Stress?* We have learned something about the microscopic appearance of injured tissue, but our view of healing phenomena is circumscribed. It is one of the profound ironies of modern medicine that we physicians are obsessed with mechanisms of injury, which are of scant interest to the sick, and glibly dismiss healing phenomena, which are of great interest to the sick. Regrettably, in clinical medicine we often deny the very existence of what we do not understand.

So it is that when we are fortunate enough to witness healing miracles—supernatural to *us*—in our practices, we reject them as figments of imagination. But there are important practical reasons why we physicians should not deny miracles, for ourselves as well as for those who trust us with their health and lives. For it is through observing what we do not understand that our understanding grows. Conversely, every time a physician rejects a miracle he witnesses, he diminishes himself.

DWARFS AND GIANTS

A dwarf standing on the shoulders of a giant may see farther than the giant himself.

Robert Burton in *The Anatomy of Melancholy*

But what if the giant is looking in the wrong direction? What would the dwarf see then?

Preface III

As I look back over my 40-years study of medicine and reflect on clinical mistakes I made myself and those I saw my colleagues make, I see something important about dwarfs, giants and enlightenment. I recognize that too many times the treating physicians were like dwarfs standing on the shoulders of the giants. Only the giants looked in the wrong direction for enlightenment. The giants of American medicine, regrettably, have been but a splendid priesthood of professionals worshipping at the altars of the gods of drugs and knives. They have been utterly committed to wiping out all competition with their chosen gods.

Unnecessary surgery was performed on a frightening scale because the giants in surgery ruthlessly suppressed effective nonsurgical options. Consider, for example, the efficacy and safety of integrated programs for reversal of coronary artery disease with optimal nutrition, meditation and chelation as opposed to the dangers and inefficacy of coronary bypass surgery.

Consider the mindless, long-term use of drugs that block essential cell receptors and cell membrane channels, inactivate core enzymes of human metabolism, suppress the immune system, destroy mediators of inflammation and healing responses, and inhibit the proton pump for necessary acid production in the stomach. There are simple, safe and effective natural therapies for most chronic nutritional, ecologic, immune and degenerative disorders that give far superior long-term clinical outcomes. But all those therapies were outlawed by the giants of drug medicine. I cite many specific examples of this pervasive phenomenon in the introduction to *RDA: Rats, Drugs and Assumptions.*

A DIFFERENT TYPE OF MEDICAL LITERATURE

True science is purity of observation. For quite some time I have recognized the need for a different type of literature. In this literature, a physician will report only what he observes himself —and not subordinate the purity of his observation to the tenets of prevailing medicine. I see a need for a new *courage* of the observing physician, a courage to state what is obvious to him regardless of how many established "principles" of medicine it violates or the giants of the field it challenges and annoys.

The different type of medical literature I refer to will not necessarily be a new type of literature. In fact, purity of clinical observation was once held in high esteem by clinicians. But then it was sacrificed on the altars of the false gods of double-blind and crossed-over studies. Whatever couldn't be blinded couldn't be trusted, so went the prevailing dogma of the giants of the drug complex. Since hope, faith, self-regulation and meditation could not be blinded, the role of such efforts in clinical medicine was dismissed as chicanery. Who benefited by such distortions in the healing profession? Who paid for such foolishness with their health and lives? The giants never permitted the dwarfs to ask such questions.

The ancients understood well what I lament here. An ancient Sanskrit text includes the following:

No matter what you hear, from whom, seeking the truth in what you hear is your wisdom.

The ancients evidently knew something about giants, dwarfs and the right direction for seeking enlightenment.

SELF-HEALING IS A DECEPTION

When humans learned to observe, they learned to self-regulate. Self-regulation took different forms in different eras and different cultures. The central observation behind it remained the same: Healing is a spontaneous phenomenon. Injured tissues heal spontaneously when they are allowed to do so. Effective methods of self-regulation and meditation allow us entry into the limbic-spiritual state (see Glossary) in which injured tissues heal spontaneously—freely and quickly. All we need to do is liberate them from the tyranny of the thinking mind.

This book describes how I, a practicing pathologist-immunologist-ecologist, entered—by destiny rather than design —the domains of self-regulation and the limbic-spiritual state. I was then unaware of the richness of the ancient writings that chronicle man's search for ways to ease his suffering and his forays into the realms of higher consciousness. I soon recognized that my clinical observations in self-regulation were of evident value to my patients. The early physical responses I observed in my patients clearly had definable electrophysiologic basis. *Those were energy events.* Those events were as real as my microscopic diagnosis of cancer and other diseases, and hence were a proper field of investigation for a physician brought up to observe physical phenomena. Anger and hostility were energy events. So were feelings of affection and love and the energy effects of the limbic-spiritual state. I was *not* into the study of consciousness then.

One simple observation in this work has influenced my thinking more than anything else: *Tissues do not lie.* So where do the distortions come from? I asked. The mind. That was the obvious answer. If the mind was the only part of the human condition that lies, why should I listen to it? This simplistic notion was reassuring. It was consistent with my years of work as an observer of microscopic events. I became intensely interested in observing electrophysiologic patterns that precede both episodes of human suffering as well as periods of relief.

VOICES OF THE INJURED TISSUES

During the years that preceded my work with self-regulation, I examined more than 50,000 biopsies of various body organs and surgical specimens. For many years I had wondered about how tissues are injured and how we pathologists name diseases. After I began my work with autoregulation, I began to wonder whether the voices we gave injured tissues were theirs or our own.

The stories of the cortical monkey and the limbic dog took shape in 1987 when I began to explore the potential of self-regulation for relieving human suffering. The two stories evolved as I described to my patients how I perceived their sufferings. Recently, Talat and I went to a Chinese restaurant. As I looked down at my soup, my eyes fell on the pictures of a monkey and a dog on the paper place mat on the table. I moved the cup of soup away and looked at the Chinese zodiac. It read:

Each of the 12 years of the Chinese zodiac falls under a different animal sign. The sign under which you were born is believed to determine the circumstances of your life and the kind of life and the kind of person you are.

Believed by who? How did the Chinese figure such things. Folklore? Myths? Why did the Chinese make such stories up to begin with? To pacify the simple-minded among them? Were these stories made by their giants for their dwarfs to serve as the opium of the masses, as the British asserted centuries later? I read along,

Monkey: Persuasive and intelligent, you strive to excel...

What a coincidence! I mused. The Chinese monkey is about

strife and persuasion, just like my cortical monkey. I read along,

Dog: Generous and loyal, you have the ability to work well with others.

The Chinese dog is about loyalty and generosity—just like my limbic dog. Another coincidence!

The Egyptians were far removed from the ancient Chinese, and they too worshipped many gods—among them, Thoth, the baboon-god who invented hieroglyphics and exhorted them to excel, just as my cortical monkey strives to excel. The cortical monkey took form before me when I saw my patients endlessly recycle past misery and—when that wasn't sufficient for them—precycle feared, future misery. The monkey of relentless thinking calculates, connives, cautions, and creates images of pain and suffering. The Chinese zodiac dog is generous and loyal. My limbic dog cares and comforts and creates images of healing. He is also generous and loyal—though he bites when confused or driven out of control by unbearable pain.

Strange coincidences!

This book is my effort to report on some extraordinary events I observed in my clinical work. It is about purity of clinical observations. I record here many of the healing miracles that the staff at the Institute and I have had the privilege of witnessing. This is my way of not letting those miracles die.

I would rather be a medical dwarf who accepts the miracles when they are told to me by my patients than be a medical giant who ridicules any healing event that he cannot comprehend simply because it cannot be controlled and blinded.

Majid Ali, M.D.
New York
March 1, 1997

Chapter 1

I Choose A Miracle

One day during my autoregulation workshop, I asked my patients if they believed in miracles. Most of them said yes enthusiastically. Some nodded tentatively. One of them shook his head and said, "No, I don't." He looked at his wife by his side, seeking her endorsement, then added, "A miracle is an outrageous thing—something that is not to be believed." Next, I asked his wife if she agreed with her husband. "I do," she spoke firmly. "Miracles are absurd events that some people imagine." Their views amused me, but I said nothing. Instead, I turned to others in the workshop. I asked them if they wanted to tell the group about events in their own lives they consider as miracles.

"What does the fellow who doesn't believe in miracles think of Newton?" Choua asked when I finished the workshop and left the autoregulation laboratory.

"Isaac Newton?" I asked, surprised. "Why Newton?"

"You should have asked him if he knows Newton discovered how a rainbow takes shape."

"Do you mean Newton's discovery of dispersion of white light into a colored spectrum? That's common knowledge. He probably does know about that."

"Does he know Newton propounded the laws of gravity,"

"That's also common knowledge. Everyone knows Newton was supposedly inspired by an apple falling to the ground. But why should I ask those question to a man who doesn't believe in miracles? I don't see what miracles have to do with gravity."

"Does he know Newton described the laws of motion?"

"What's on your mind, Choua?" I asked, a trifle irritated. "That man said he thinks miracles are absurd. I don't see what miracles have to do with rainbow colors or with the laws of gravity and motion."

"Does he know Newton also developed differential calculus?" he went on, ignoring my question.

"Why should I care whether he does or doesn't know about Newton's differential calculus? What does calculus have to do with miracles anyway?" I asked, my irritation growing.

"Does he think Newton was one of the greatest mathematicians and physicists who ever lived?" he again ignored my question.

"What's your point, Choua?" I asked sternly. "Where is this inquiry taking us?"

"Does he agree Newton was one of the most brilliant intellects in the history of science?" he asked calmly.

"I think you made your point," I snapped. "Newton was a great scientist. Every child in school knows that. But we were talking about miracles, not science. Weren't we?"

"You should have asked him if Newton would have found the idea of humans flying 40,000 feet above the ground outrageous."

"What?" I was taken aback.

"Yes. He dismisses miracles as outrageous things. You should have asked him if the discoverer of gravity and laws of motion could have imagined how supersonic jets might fly," he goaded me with a smile.

"Could Newton have foreseen the invention of the Concorde? Is that the question?" I asked, puzzled.

"Yes. Yes." Choua chirped. "You should have asked him if Newton would have considered the notion of someone flying from London to New York in three hours an outrageous thing, something not to be believed."

"Oh! That!" The words slipped from my lips.

"Yes, that!" He grinned impishly, then continued, "What is an outrageous proposition for one can be a simple and observable phenomenon for another."

"But you could have said all that in one short sentence," I taunted. "You didn't have to bring gravity, mechanics and rainbows into that."

"In 1714 the British Parliament enacted the Longitude Act, and promised a prize of 20,000 pounds to any one who invented a clock that would carry the true time from the home port to remote seas of the world," he went on calmly. "Did you know that Newton feared that the task was impossible?"

"No, I didn't until you enlightened me just this moment," I replied, exasperated.

"Tell me about James." Choua abruptly changed the subject.

"James who?" I asked, puzzled.

"Tell me about James," he repeated. "Tell me about the miracle of his heart. He received one coronary bypass operation in 1984 and was told he needed another in 1987. Tell me about what happened next."

"What's there to tell? You know all about him."

"Tell me anyway," he pressed.

A MIRACLE OF THE HEART

I first saw James K. in 1987. He looked tired, distraught and frightened. After he sat on a chair, he looked at me nervously, then at his wife on the next chair, and finally down at his feet. His wife gave me a brief history of his illness. James had suffered advanced coronary artery disease for several years. In 1984 he underwent a bypass that evidently had failed. He had daily angina attacks and heart palpitations that were not relieved by the multiple drug therapies his cardiologist had prescribed. On many days he couldn't walk up the stairs to his bedroom, so he slept downstairs. Finally, his cardiologist told him that even though the possibility of success with a second bypass operation was less than 20 percent, he still urged James to consider it because the cardiologist didn't see an alternative. James emphatically declined the second bypass operation.

During his initial consultation with me, James's wife left the room for a few moments. James looked at the closed door behind her and spoke in clear, firm words, "Dr. Ali, I had a bypass three years ago that didn't work. I suffer angina every day. I'm homebound now. I have no life. They tell me I need another bypass operation and that there isn't much chance of its success. I don't want any heroics now. Everyone has to go some day. I want to leave with dignity." I told him I fully respected his views. When his wife returned to the consultation room, she told me she was hoping I would immediately begin EDTA chelation therapy.

I had only recently passed the examination for the diploma of the American Board of Chelation Therapy. My clinical experience with such therapy had been limited, and I wasn't yet clear about its clinical benefits. EDTA chelation was then—and regrettably continues to be—a highly controversial therapy for coronary artery disease. Most cardiologists dismiss it as sheer chicanery. I knew only too well the dangers to my professional reputation as well as to my medical license for trying a controversial therapy with a critically ill patient. It seemed to me a plainly foolish proposition for an inexperienced physician to try to tackle a case of advanced coronary artery disease. I was very conscious of my limitations. James's case evidently was considered extremely serious by his cardiologist. I wasn't about to jump into therapy for a patient that I had hardly met when I knew his experienced cardiologist was extremely pessimistic. There were also the critical issues of informed consent and legally valid documentation of the true state of affairs.

James's wife quickly sensed my reticence and began to plead her husband's case. "We'll do anything you say. We'll follow your program fully. If you're concerned about legal issues, we'll sign any consent you want." I tried to be as gentle as I could in presenting to them my reasons for not taking the case. I told them I could refer them to Robert Atkins, M.D., in New York who I knew was experienced in EDTA chelation therapy and also well-versed with all issues of such therapy for advanced coronary artery disease. Both she and James adamantly refused that. Next, I suggested some names of New Jersey physicians who offered chelation services. The more I recommended other physicians, the more she insisted I take the case. I held my ground.

Finally she said, "Dr. Ali, we live only a few blocks from your office. Please do what you can. Please give him some chelation. He's the only husband I have." Weakened by their persistence and utterly against my better judgment, I agreed to treat James. I emphasized the need for a full clinical evaluation with focus on stress reduction and optimal kitchen choices. And after James's clinical situation was stabilized, I explained further, I would recommend slow, limbic exercise.

EDTA chelation therapy worked extremely well for James. The frequency of chest pain episodes and heart palpitations diminished. After some months of treatment, he began to go out for walks. After some more months of clinical improvement, I began to taper his drug doses and to discontinue some of them. About eight years later, during a follow-up visit in February 1994, I asked James how many heart drugs he was taking. He replied that he then took one-half of one heart pill—on alternate days. Curious about what possible benefits there could be in taking such a small drug dose, I asked him why he did that. "I'm superstitious," he replied with a disarming smile. "Keep it up,

James," I counseled.

In the spring of 1995, James developed a severe chest pain while defending himself against some vandals. He landed in the ICU of Mountainside Hospital near our Bloomfield office. His cardiology team checked him inside and out over a period of five days and found no evidence of coronary artery disease.

About ten years after beginning our integrated program for reversing coronary artery disease—including optimal food choices, nutrient and herbal therapies, autoregulation, limbic exercise and EDTA chelation—James is now free of angina pains and heart palpitations. From time to time he experiences momentary tightness in his chest muscles, which he controls with limbic breathing. He walks three miles a day and hasn't touched a heart drug in almost two years.

"James was a cardiac cripple when you first saw him," Choua spoke after I finished telling him the case history. "His story had a good clinical outcome. Right?"

"It's more than a good clinical outcome, Choua," I replied. "It is most extraordinary. Indeed, it is unbelievable."

"Would you have believed it if anyone had told you that *total* reversal of advanced coronary artery disease was possible in a person judged irreversible by his cardiologist?"

"It would have been difficult. His cardiologist did not hold out much hope for him. I told you he was ready to call it quits."

"His coronary disease was considered terminal by his cardiologist. Right?"

"Right."

"How does he look back at those days of being a cardiac cripple?"

"Sometimes I ask him about that nightmare. He tries to

avoid the subject of bypass surgery."

"Too traumatic?"

"Yes. I suggested to him several times that he get a thallium heart scan to see how well his heart muscle is supplied with blood now, but he finds the very idea of seeing a cardiologist traumatic. So I don't push him anymore."

"What exactly did he say when you asked him to see a cardiologist for a thallium scan?" he asked impishly.

"He said the word cardiologist gives him cardiac spasms."

"Suppose his cardiologist had been told that ten years after he pronounced James's heart problem irremediable, he would be free of angina and heart palpitations. Do you think he would have believed it?"

"I don't think so."

"If you hadn't followed James's case personally for all those years, wouldn't you have found James's case history an absurd proposition?"

"Yes."

"How many cardiologists would still find it an absurd proposition?"

"Some. Many. Well, I really don't know," I faltered.

"Suppose someone had told you ten years ago that chelation and nutrient therapies would reverse James's coronary artery disease. Would you have believed it?"

"No."

"What would you choose to call James's case history?" Choua's voice fell into a murmur. "Is it an absurd proposition? Or a case of anecdotal spontaneous healing? Or a miracle?"

"I choose a miracle." The words slipped from my lips before I realized what I had said.

Choua laughed. He has a way of turning and twisting my words, then using them effectively against me. On most occasions

I would have fought back. But James is my favorite patient. More than any other patient, he changed my entire perspective on the reversibility of advanced coronary heart disease—or the irreversibility of the lesions, as most cardiologists continue to insist on calling it. It was impossible for me to rebuke Choua, no matter how much I wanted to, while he made his case using James's case history. I laughed as well.

A MIRACLE OF A PLACEBO

On November 12, 1996, I presented the results of our above-cited EDTA chelation study at Holy Name Hospital, Teaneck, New Jersey. I first presented that study in 1994 at the annual meeting of the American Academy of Preventive Medicine in New York. I include an abstract of that study at the end of this chapter. In that study my colleagues and I reported an excellent outcome (defined as 100% control of symptoms as well as complete discontinuance of all drugs) in 61% of the patients with advanced coronary artery disease. In another 17%, the outcome was deemed good (defined as more than 75% reduction in symptoms as well as drug dosage). The clinical outcome in 13% of the study subjects was considered moderately successful (defined as 50% reduction in symptoms as well as drug dose reduction). Only one patient reported no clinical benefit from EDTA chelation. Those were astonishing results and most physicians, in fact, would find them too good to be true.

At Holy Name, however, I was at a significant advantage. Most of the physicians in the audience knew me well. I had served as the Director of the Departments of Pathology, Immunology and

Laboratories in the hospital for over two decades. Most of the audience also knew one of my co-investigators, Alfred O. Fayemi, M.D. I knew our data wouldn't be rejected simply because it seemed too good to be true.

There was a question-answer session after my presentation. Most questions concerned aspects of chelation therapy that I hadn't covered due to time constraints. A young internist challenged the validity of our study on the grounds that we had not established any controls for patients in the study. Before I could answer, an older internist intervened and spoke about the infeasibility and the ethical problem of administering placebo drips to seriously ill patients who couldn't be helped with coronary bypass surgery, angioplasty and extensive drug therapies. The young internist was unsatisfied with the explanation of the older physician. He shook his head in disapproval and muttered something about the placebo effect and the absolute need for the controls and rigors of science.

After the conference I was scheduled to see some patients in my office. I decided not to engage that young internist in a debate that I considered futile. The very notion of keeping very sick patients in the blind while I administered placebo infusions was repugnant to me. Does this young physician really understand what he is saying? I wondered. All of our patients in the study suffered from documented, advanced, life-threatening heart disease. Coronary bypass operations, angioplasties and drug therapies had failed. How could any one of us ever give one half of them plain salt water as a placebo so that we could satisfy the critics?

"Do you think the young internist understood that your patients were failures of angioplasterers, coronary bypass technicians and the drug specialists?" Choua asked as I left the conference hall.

"I'm sure he understood that," I replied, ignoring his sarcasm. "I think he was troubled that we didn't have a proper control group and that our clinical results could have all been due to the placebo effect of the EDTA therapy," I replied.

"Ah, the placebo effect of EDTA!" Choua smirked. "He is young and can be forgiven for his disdain of the placebo effect. When he grows older, he will learn to love the placebo effect of chelation therapy too."

"Love the placebo effect?" I asked, puzzled.

"Oh yes! He'll learn to love the placebo effect of EDTA chelation therapy as I do," he grinned.

"You're not serious, are you?"

"Isn't it marvelous that the miracle of the placebo effect of EDTA worked where the science and statistics of coronary bypass surgery had miserably failed?" he asked with a wink.

"I suppose you can say that." I suppressed a smile.

"And isn't it wonderful that the placebo effects of EDTA restored health for the seriously ill for whom the science and statistics of coronary angioplasty brought no relief?"

"Right."

"And isn't it splendid that the placebo of EDTA worked where the science and statistics of drug therapies failed?"

"Right again."

"Suppose that young internist himself were to suffer from advanced coronary artery disease and the placebo effects of angioplasty, coronary bypass surgery and drug therapies failed to relieve his suffering. Do you think he would still ridicule the placebo of EDTA chelation therapy if his life depended on it as did the lives of patients in your study?"

"You're a rascal." I couldn't control my laughter.

A PRESCRIPTION FOR SPIRITUAL SURRENDER

"How do we know how much of the benefit was due to EDTA chelation and how much was due to other components of our total program?" I asked after a while.

"What components?" he asked.

"Nutrition, exercise and spiritual work."

"It's not as difficult as you make it to be."

"Maybe it isn't difficult for you, but it is for me."

"What's the greatest danger patients with advanced coronary artery disease face?"

"A spasm of a coronary artery that can completely cut off all circulation to the heart muscle and cause a fatal heart attack."

"Is there a food that can halt a coronary artery spasm?"

"I don't know of any."

"Is there a type of exercise that can halt a severe coronary artery spasm?"

"There's none. Indeed, any exercise during an intense coronary spasm can prove fatal. So that would be very dangerous."

"Is there a prayer that can do it?"

"Aha! Now you're coming close to the real thing. Prayer can be the best defense against a life-threatening spasm."

"How often do you see highly stressed coronary patients in real life who can suddenly learn a prayer that quickly dissolves coronary spasms?"

"That's a real problem. To relieve coronary artery spasm, one needs to learn to surrender to that larger *presence* that permeates and surrounds each of us. And that takes diligent work—it takes years of training. You can't get that sort of ability on short order."

"In other words, you can't give a patient a prescription for spiritual surrender. It doesn't work that way, does it?"

"No. It doesn't."

"There! That's the answer to your question," Choua chuckled. "EDTA is a powerful coronary spasm buster. It is an effective blood thinner. It is a potent cell membrane stabilizer. And, of course, it's a major antioxidant. That's the critical role of EDTA in the early months of therapy."

Choua had made his case persuasively. There was nothing there for me to refute. I kept quiet. I thought about the many times I had heard cardiologists at the hospital ridicule chelation doctors. At that time I had no firsthand knowledge of the potential of EDTA chelation therapy for preventing deaths from heart disease.

Regrettably, most cardiologists continue to dismiss chelation therapy as unproven. Without taking the time to study patients who have been managed with this approach, they make irresponsible statements against it. To my knowledge, in *RDA: Rats, Drugs and Assumptions,* I published the first color pictures of pre- and post-treatment thallium scans of the heart, conclusively proving the efficacy of our integrated program for reversing advanced coronary artery disease, including EDTA chelation therapy. At the time of this writing, we have obtained several pairs of pre- and post-chelation scans. To date, 90% of such scans show objective evidence of positive results obtained with EDTA chelation therapy. I devote the companion volume, *Cholesterol Cats, Chelation Mice and the Heart* to this subject.

A MIRACLE OF A BRAIN TUMOR

"What is a malignant glioma?" Choua asked.

"It's a highly aggressive brain cancer," I replied.

"Can it be controlled by surgery?"

"No. The problem is, it freely invades the surrounding brain tissue. So neurosurgeons look at the tumor, take a biopsy and close the skull. They know they have no chance of complete removal."

"Does radiotherapy work for it?"

"Malignant gliomas are considered radio-resistant."

"Does chemotherapy work for it?"

"No."

"Do oncologists treat such cancers with chemotherapy?"

"Sometimes."

"Why? If they know chemo doesn't work for gliomas, why do they do it?"

"I've heard some oncologists say they do it for its anecdotal value."

"Anecdotal value?" Choua's eyes narrowed. "Isn't the use of nutritional therapies for anecdotal value considered quackery by drug doctors?"

"The first time I heard an oncologist say that in a conference, I was just as surprised as you are," I replied.

"Interesting!" Choua chuckled. "I guess the use of toxic chemo drugs for known chemo-resistant cancers is okay for their anecdotal values but the use of nontoxic nutrient therapies for their anecdotal value isn't. Drug doctors do have their own way of rationalizing drug therapies."

"That's a terrible mistake," I agreed.

"Last night you saw a woman in her sixties who developed a malignant glioma in 1994. During surgery, her tumor was found too extensive to be completely removed. The neurosurgeon biopsied the tumor and closed the wound. She was administered radiation therapy, even though radiation is known to be ineffective against malignant gliomas. How long was she given to live?"

"She was given three months to live. She said her sister forbade her neurosurgeon to tell her about her prognosis. The neurosurgeon protested, saying that it was against New Jersey state law. Her sister replied indignantly, 'That may be against New Jersey law. But we're from Tennessee. And that's not against Tennessee law.'"

"How did she find out about the prognosis?"

"I asked her about it. She smiled and said, 'My sister told me about the surgeon's time limit on my life two years later when the repeat scans showed no evidence of a tumor in my head.'"

"What do you think of that?"

"Hard to believe. I was just as astonished at her recovery, as was her neurosurgeon, and as you are now."

"What would you choose to call it?" he winked impishly. "Is that case history an absurd proposition? A deception? An irritating anecdote for drug doctors who scoff at notions of supernatural events? Or was that a miracle?"

"I choose a miracle."

A MIRACLE OF MULTIPLE SCLEROSIS

"David G. suffered from multiple sclerosis (MS) and couldn't walk one half of a city block without falling when he first saw you," Choua resumed. "You remember him, don't you?"

"How could I ever forget him?" I answered. "That's another incredible case history."

"Tell me, what did the MRI scan of the head show?"
"Multiple white lesions that indicated MS."
"What causes those white lesions?"
"Loss of the myelin sheath—a thin layer of fatty substances that insulates nerve fibers and prevents short-circuiting."
"What causes the loss of myelin sheath?"
"Autoimmune injury."
"What causes autoimmune injury?"
"In mainstream medical thinking, the cause of autoimmune injury is not known."
"What do you think is the cause?"
"Mold allergy and mycotoxin toxicity, food allergy, metabolic immune suppression, chemical and heavy metal toxicity. And when the immune defenses are broken, chronic viral activation syndromes develop."
"How is David doing now? How is he walking?"
"That's remarkable. Today, more than five years after I first saw him, he walks miles without any leg instability. He has none of the other MS symptoms, such as skin numbness and burning, muscle spasms and urinary problems. I haven't seen him in two years, but I know one of his good friends who tells me that he is doing very well."
"Hard to believe. Tell me about his current brain MRI scans."
"That's even more amazing. His scans are now completely normal. There's no sign of any white MS lesions."
"Would you say his MS has been reversed?"
"So far, so good, but you know MS is a disease characterized by relapses and remissions. I don't take that outcome as proof of a cure, and I pray that he continues to be free of

problems of multiple sclerosis*. I wish it could be that simple for my other MS patients, and that I could promise such results to everyone with this disorder, but it isn't..."

"I'm not talking about other patients," he interrupted me abruptly. "Let's stay with David's case. Would you choose to call his case history an absurd proposition? Something not to be believed? A rare case of anecdotal spontaneous resolution? Or would you choose to call it a miracle?"

"I choose a miracle," I confessed.

"The wife of the man we spoke of earlier rejects miracles as absurd events that some people imagine," Choua resumed. "You should have asked her if she has read about Nicolaus Copernicus."

"Why should I have asked her questions about Copernicus?" I inquired. Then, realizing what Choua was up to, I added, "You're not going through another Newton story, are you?"

"Copernicus was a gifted man. He observed the position of planets in the sky and figured out that the ancient Egyptians were wrong. He believed that the Ptolemaic notion, that all heavenly bodies moved around the earth was in error. He was convinced the earth revolved around the sun."

"So?"

"Does that woman think Copernicus would have believed a document could be sent from Denville to Denmark in seconds?"

---

* I have discussed in detail the management of severe autoimmune disorders, such as multiple sclerosis, in the companion volume *The Canary and Chronic Fatigue*. Here, I list the essentials of such a program: limbic-spiritual work; overhydration during daytime hours; optimal nutrient and herbal therapies; management of mold and food allergies; restoration of the bowel, blood, and other body organ ecosystems; normalization of hormonal status; hydrotherapies; colon therapies; and slow, nongoal-oriented limbic exercise.

"Oh no!" I laughed. "You're not going to repeat that whole thing now, are you?"

"Copernicus was a brilliant man. Ask her if he would have accepted the plausibility of a fax machine."

"Probably not." I conceded, suppressing a smile.

"Ask her if twenty years ago she would have rejected as absurd the possibility of transmitting reams of paper over phone lines," he grinned and bared his teeth. "Then ask her..."

"Okay! Okay! You made your point," I cut him off. "But that's all hard science."

"Galileo Galilei discovered four satellites of Jupiter with his telescope and told people that Copernicus was right after all. Then he...?"

"Wait! Wait! Choua," I interrupted him, piqued by his obsessive raving. "Keep Galileo out of this. I really don't want a lesson in the history of astronomy. I don't know what all that stuff has to do with miracles."

"Poor Galileo was born at the wrong time and in the wrong country. Newton was born the year Galileo died, in 1642. And Newton was an Englishman."

"Look, Choua, science is science and miracles are miracles. I don't know why you're dragging Newton and Galileo into this discussion," I protested.

"The Italians persecuted poor Galileo mercilessly, and the Pope forced him to recant," he went on, ignoring my protest. "Newton might have met a similar fate had he not been more circumspect. But he knew better than to blend science with his interest in theology."

"Newton never got into trouble with the clergy, did he?" I asked, surprised.

"Not with the clergy, but with the British monarchy. During his later years, he was preoccupied with the interpretation of prophesies and other theological works, even though people only knew about his later editions of *Principia* and *Opticks*. In 1716 Caroline, Princess of Wales, heard about his new principles of chronology and asked him to produce a copy for her. That was a double jeopardy. He dared not refuse the princess's order, yet he couldn't risk her wrath by revealing his heretical assertions."

"What did he do then?" I asked, my curiosity piqued.

"That was his master stroke. He begged her for a few days to complete his chronology and penned a 'Short Chronology' from which he excluded all materials that he thought might offend the royals. You see, Newton knew Galileo's fate, and he wasn't about to let his science tangle with the clergy or royalty."

"Okay, okay, Choua. Now what does all this have to do with miracles?" I asked curtly, returning to the subject.

"What is a miracle?" Choua asked with a frown.

"Some people define miracles as supernatural events —happenings that are beyond the laws of nature," I replied.

"What are the laws of nature?" he shot back.

"The physical laws of nature, such as the pull of the earth's gravity and Newton's laws of motion." I felt uneasy as soon as Newton's name slipped through my lips.

"Who defines the laws of nature?" Choua asked, a knowing smile spreading on his face.

"Physicists and biologists, chemists and..."

"Then they disagree among themselves and change *their* laws of nature, don't they?" he mocked.

"Give me an example," I contested.

"Newton thought his armor had no chinks. Einstein looked for them and found some. At high velocities and large gravities, Newtonian physics doesn't hold."

"Well, Newton lived a long time ago. I don't think that sort of thing happens anymore."

"No?" he growled. "Hydrogen is the simplest of elements. For decades, chemists have taught that hydrogen atoms are always positively charged. Now they have changed their mind. They teach us that in certain molecules, such as amine borane, hydrogen atoms have a negative charge. That was reported in the July 1996 issue of *Accounts of Chemical Research.* But, why should such a thing surprise you? Don't you read *Science* and *Nature* every month?"

This was the first time I learned that hydrogen atoms can be negatively charged. I decided not to say anything.

MEDICINE AND MIRACLES DON'T MIX

"Why don't you doctors like miracles?" Choua asked.
"It's not a matter of liking or disliking," I replied.
"What's it about then?"
"Medicine and miracles don't mix," I replied.
"Who said that?" Choua turned sharply and stared me in the eyes.
"Everyone says that," I replied lamely.
"Who is everyone?"
"Professors in medical schools. Researchers in laboratories."
"Who else?"
"Scientists in chemistry and biology labs."
"Who else?"
"Engineers and lawyers and judges."
"That's an impressive list," he commented.
"What's the point of this inquiry?" I asked, annoyed.
"A question arises before a scientist. For years he diligently seeks an answer to his riddle. One day he hypothesizes about the

solution to that riddle. Some time later he makes a physical observation that validates his hypothesis. That observation is accepted by many, but not all, as valid proof of the hypothesis. Right?"

"Yes, that often happens."

"What would you call that?"

"Where is that leading us?" I asked, vexed by his rambling dialogue.

"A question arises before a mystic," he went on without acknowledging my frustration. "For years he also diligently seeks an answer to his riddle. One day he hypothesizes about the solution to his riddle. Some time later he makes an observation with his inward eye that validates his hypothesis. That observation is accepted by many, but not all, as valid proof for the hypothesis. Tell me, what's the difference between what the open eyes of the scientist see and what the closed eyes of the mystic discern?"

"That's preposterous!" I retorted angrily. "There is a world of difference between the two. The physical observation made by the open eyes of the scientist is for anyone to test—and validate or refute. Who knows what the closed eyes of the mystic see? How can you speak about the two in the same breath?"

"Ah, the closed eye of the mystic," Choua's voice fell to a murmur as he continued, his eyes slowly closing. "What does the open eye of the scientist observe? What does the unopened eye of the mystic see? And what's the difference between the two? And what about when the open eye cannot see?"

Choua stood motionless, his eyes closed, receding from my presence. I looked at him and wondered what his cryptic words meant to him. What does the unopened eye of the mystic see? I wanted to ask him to explain himself, but decided not to. Several minutes passed.

"Do you remember when Kim's mom rushed Kim into your office with an asthma attack?" he asked finally, slowly opening his eyes.

"What does asthma have to do with what a mystic's unopened eye might or might not see?" I asked. "I've never heard of a mystic who was interested in inhaler therapy for asthma."

Choua grinned, then looked away. He suffers from attention deficit disorder and often has a great deal of difficulty staying focused on the subject under discussion. On most days I overlook his handicap. Sometimes I am amused by his wandering mind; at other times I am baffled by it. Then there are days when I know that talking to him means punishing myself. There is no order to his words—no specific beginning, no discrete ending. Still, it is hard to disentangle myself. On that day he shifted from one subject to another in his schizophrenic flight of ideas. What does a mystic's unopened eye have to do with Kim's asthma? And what do asthma and mysticism together have to do with miracles? I wondered.

THE MIRACLE IN A CHEMISTRY LAB

"That's some thought dissociation, Choua," I mocked. "But tell me, what does Kim's asthma have to do with the mystic's inward eye? Can you speak plainly for once?"

"You remember Kim's asthma attack, don't you?" he asked, then added, "She was blue in the face and gasped for breath with all her energy."

My thoughts drifted to Kim, a pretty six-year-old, who

suffers from asthma. Choua was referring to the day when I saw Kim's mom rush into our office, carrying her daughter in her arms. Kim was wheezing loudly and gasping for breath. Her face was blue from lack of oxygen, and I could see her ribs struggle each time she pulled at them to breathe. She had developed an acute asthma attack during her car trip to our office. Once in the office, her mother calmly opened her handbag, pulled out an inhaler and a collapsed breathing bag, prepared the bag, and put it on her daughter's face. Minutes later, the little girl's face turned pink. Kim removed the bag from her face, looked at me, and broke out in an enchanting smile. I patted her head, relieved and happy for her.

"The drug in Kim's inhaler worked well, didn't it?" Choua's voice brought me back.

"Yes, it did," I replied. "The inhaler broke Kim's bronchial spasm so she could breathe."

"The drug was a synthetic molecule, wasn't it?"

"Yes, it was."

"That synthetic drug didn't exist in nature until some chemist *witnessed* its creation in a test tube. Right?"

"Right!" I conceded.

"What laws of nature did that synthetic drug follow?"

"What do you mean?"

"A seventeenth-century physician would have considered it supernatural for someone to create a substance in his laboratory that could break a severe asthma attack in minutes. Right?"

"Probably yes."

"Then a miracle took place in a chemist's laboratory. A molecule came into being that can halt an asthma attack. Right?" he smiled mysteriously.

"Yes! No! I mean..." I stammered. "But science requires diligent research."

"That's not what I asked about," he said acidly.

"Who knows what you ramble about," I said, miffed by the sudden change in his tone.

"So, did or didn't that chemist's drug perform a miracle? Is that a yes or a no?" Choua was unrelenting.

"I might argue that the synthesis of that drug molecule was still following some law of chemistry that brings many atoms together to make a new compound." I refused to yield.

"That's not what I mean." He frowned.

"Who knows what you mean?" I snapped. "Why can't we say that nature created the chemist who, in turn, created the drug in accordance with the laws of nature? Isn't that what synthetic chemistry is all about?"

"Don't you see?" Choua groused. "Before the drug was synthesized, and before its clinical efficacy was established by research, the asthma-breaking action of that drug was not a part of the *then* known laws of nature."

"It may not have been known to some, but it was there to be discovered," I held my ground.

"Aha!" he erupted. "I was hoping you would say that. Do you ever wonder how many more such laws of nature still *remain to be discovered?*" His eyes narrowed. "How many miracles of today that you dismiss as absurd will prove to be entirely logical and predictable in years to come?"

I felt a growing uneasiness with the conversation. I couldn't agree with Choua and yet found it difficult to disagree. We all know what miracles are, I thought. Or at least I thought I knew what they were—events that appear unexplainable by the laws of nature and so are held to be supernatural in origin. Miracles are acts of God that humans will never understand, that's what I had been told many years earlier. Now here was Choua enunciating a new, tangled theory of miracles which I could neither accept nor reject. I looked at him in silence. He stared back at me for several moments, then spoke in low measured tones.

ONLY THE PROFOUNDLY IGNORANT DENY MIRACLES

"We're still left with the core problem," Choua resumed. "Who decides what the laws of nature are today? And who decides what the laws of nature will be tomorrow? And the day after? How many of the supernatural wonders of yesteryear are *entirely natural* today? How many of the things that you consider supernatural today—absurd propositions that are not to be heeded, as that man and his wife put it—will be accepted as completely natural in years to come?"

"Well, in that sense, every scientific discovery, every technical advance is a miracle," I remarked.

"I'd hoped you'd see that." His eyes lit up.

"But isn't that playing with words?"

"Playing with words?" he snarled. "I'm dead serious. And you should be too."

"Take it easy," I chided Choua. "It's just a conversation."

"How many of your colleagues in drug medicine snicker at their patients when they talk about miracles?" he growled. "How many of them revile people who might admit the possibility of miracles in clinical medicine? And then how many of the same miracle-bashing drug doctors excitedly talk about their miracle drugs?"

"Well, that..."

"So the drug miracles are kosher for drug doctors, but nutrient miracles aren't. Is that it?" he gored.

"What's eating you today?" I retorted.

Choua opened his mouth to say something, then seemed to change his mind and rubbed his temple. I knew he was not finished with his diatribe against people who deny the possibility of miracles. I welcomed the respite from his barrage of questions, but knew that it wouldn't last long. After some minutes, he resumed in a low tone:

"Only the profoundly ignorant deny the possibility of miracles."

"That's a strong statement, Choua. What do you mean?" I asked.

"You say a miracle is a supernatural event. How does anyone know what supernatural is?"

"That's simple enough! Supernatural is something beyond the natural. I think every reasonable person would agree to that."

"Not that simple!" he countered. "Before you can consider anything beyond *something*, you must first know what *that something* is. Right?"

"Go on."

"Before you declare an event supernatural, you must first be certain that you know *all* of what nature is. Now tell me who can be so arrogant to stake that kind of a claim except the profoundly ignorant?"

"You do have a way with words, Choua," I taunted. "You can find a way to ridicule anything you want."

"Not anything! Only what needs to be ridiculed."

"Okay! Okay! I concede. What next?"

A DIFFERENT VIEW OF THE MIRACLE

Choua was forcing me to look at miracles in an altogether different way. He had deftly cited case histories that I couldn't refute. But there's more to clinical medicine than that, I thought. I see patients with advanced coronary artery disease and failed bypass operations and angioplasties every day. Most of those patients do very well with our total program including EDTA chelation therapy. Still, can I promise superb results like those we witnessed with James to everyone with advanced heart disease?

David recovered completely from multiple sclerosis. His MRI scan is completely free of MS lesions. Can I tell my other MS patients his success story? And, my God, what wouldn't I do if I could help all my other MS patients dissolve their brain lesions the way David did? The woman with highly malignant glioma beat all the odds. Every working day, I see patients with advanced, widespread cancer. But they don't tell me about their triumphs as did the woman with malignant glioma of the brain.

Choua is right. But he is also wrong. Where is he wrong? I wondered. Can I tell every new heart patient James's story? Can such hope be sustained in each case? What would happen if some patients showed poor results? What would be the true cost of the shattered hopes in such an individual? Can I tell every new MS patient David's case history? Wouldn't that be cruel to many people who might not recover? Is it responsible for me to tell patients with brain cancers the story of the woman from Tennessee? Would that be ethical? And what would happen when those hopes are not fulfilled? How does one cope with that kind of disillusionment? And pain? And anguish? How does a physician face the young children of a woman who succumbs to breast cancer? How does he cope with the family left behind by a man dying of prostate cancer? When is hope healing? When does it become a cruel deception? How does one know the difference between the two?

THE MYSTERY OF HEALING DEEPENS

"There are good reasons for believing in miracles," Choua resumed, "both from the doctor's as well as the patient's perspective."

"What?" I asked indifferently, still caught in my private struggle.

"The possibility of miracles forces the doctor to recognize his *very* limited understanding of healing."

"And for the very ill patient?"

"Believing in miracles allows the patient to defy his doctor's prognosis and create his own reservoir of hope."

"That would be wonderful if it were to happen," I said, more to respond than to really participate in the conversation. I was too engrossed with my inward dialogue.

As a hospital pathologist for 29 years, I had studied more than 100,000 surgical specimens. We pathologists can recognize the healing process taking place in injured tissues. But when it comes to explaining the energetic-molecular phenomena that trigger the healing, we're at a loss.

How does a cell at the edge of a surgeon's incision know that its neighboring cell has been cut through so it must now respond to the call of the injured cell? How do the cells lining tiny capillaries at the edges of the sutured incisions know that they must now multiply and send delicate tendrils into the coagulum of plasma that fills the narrow space between the wound margins? When a person bleeds after an auto accident, how do the parent cells in the bone marrow know they have to multiply to make up for the lost cells? Perhaps there are hormones that stimulate cells in the marrow. How do those hormones know that they have to carry different messages after blood loss? Indeed, how do the cells that produce those hormones know they need to produce them?

The fact is, the more we explore the mystery of healing, the deeper it becomes. Our inquiry only reveals how little we truly know.

INJURED CELLS DON'T LIE: THE MIRACLE OF OBSERVATION

"This week you saw Debbie. Her mother told you she had tried to commit suicide several weeks ago and had been hospitalized for several days. Then she was discharged on Prozac. Her mother was frightened out of her wits because Debbie had not taken Prozac for nine days and was sinking deeper into depression. She had refused to see her psychiatrist or pediatrician. Before she left your office, she agreed to take her Prozac. Tell me, how did that happen?"

"You're bringing up one miraculous case history after another, Choua. But that can be very misleading. You know we don't succeed in all cases like that," I replied.

"Go ahead. Humor me," he prodded. "Tell me about Debbie anyway."

I told Choua about the extraordinary visit I had with 15-year-old Debbie. Her mother had wanted to see me alone before I saw Debbie. During the interview, she told me how worried she was and pleaded hard for help. It was evident from the questionnaire she had completed that Debbie was an allergic child, but her allergies were never diagnosed. She suffered from frequent throat and ear infections as a child, for which she was prescribed many antibiotics. When she grew up she was given yet more antibiotics for acne and other skin infections. She also suffered from wild mood swings. However, depression was not a part of her clinical picture until she turned 13.

When Debbie entered my office with her mother, she kept her eyes fixed on the floor. I tried to bring her out of her melancholy with different lines of questioning, but to no avail. Then I directed my questions to her mother. Each time her mother answered my questions, I studied Debbie's face for some clue as to how I might lift the dark curtains of her anguish. There were no signs. More than half an hour into the visit, it became apparent I had no chance of breaking through to her. I began explaining to the mother that I wasn't set up to provide care for seriously depressed persons like Debbie. Then I felt an impulse and did something I had never done before with a depressed patient. I asked Debbie if she would let me have a sample drop of her blood from a finger stick. To my amazement, she nodded her head. Maybe I can connect, I murmured to myself.

I made a smear of a drop of Debbie's blood on a slide and placed it on the stage of my high-resolution microscope equipped with phase-contrast and dark-field optics. Then I picked up my album of color pictures of blood morphology studies and began to show Debbie various patterns of oxidative injury to blood cells and plasma proteins in fresh blood. She showed no interest. I showed her yet more pictures of damaged and disfigured red blood cells and immune cells. I pointed out clumps of bacteria, yeast and various types of synthetic junk that I often see floating in the bloodstream. Debbie stole a few glimpses but remained sad and indifferent. It was then that I turned the microscope light on, switched on the video attached to my microscope, shook her blood smear slide a little to dramatize the motion of blood cells, and said, suddenly raising the tone of my voice, "Look, Debbie, now I have your blood on the video. Let's see what we can find." Debbie stiffened, then tentatively looked at the video screen. I knew then that Debbie was hooked—it was the break I'd been waiting for.

I wrote in *The Cortical Monkey and Healing* that the only part of the human condition that lies is the mind. The blood, heart, skin and muscles never lie. I'd seen on numerous occasions how simple observations of one's own biology—whether seen as the moving graph lines of the heart function obtained with electrophysiologic sensors or as color pictures of one's own blood ecosystem—can profoundly alter a person's perception of health and disease. Biologic profiles, such as the one I showed to Debbie that day don't lie. Debbie's blood revealed a lot to me—and to Debbie—as I slowly and gently pointed out the various abnormalities in her cells and microclots of plasma proteins to her. A majority of her red blood cells were deformed and stuck to each other, causing extensive sludging—a phenomenon that impairs the flow of blood in capillaries, including those in the brain. As I scanned her smear, most of the video screens showed microclots of plasma proteins, indicating excessive oxidative denaturation of her blood proteins. Innumerable yeast organisms were readily seen. It was an impressive display of changes that would have moved anyone. And so it moved Debbie.

Next, I explained to Debbie the causes of her blood abnormalities, and outlined my global plan for reversing the damage done to her blood cells and plasma with nondrug nutrient and herbal therapies. I furthermore explained that the drop of her blood, which we looked at, was in reality a window to her biology, and it reflected changes in all her cells and tissue fluids. Debbie was now a captive of the microscope. Her eyes remained glued to the video screen. I returned to my album and showed her how we had reversed similar abnormalities in other patients.

Finally, I looked Debbie in the eye and said, "Debbie, please listen to me carefully. I'm going to say something that you or your mom may not like. If so, you may simply wish to stand up and leave the room. No hard feelings. I am a physician who believes there is a physical basis for every suffering, and that there is no such nonsense as psychiatric illness. I know you have a different neurochemistry that makes you very sad. But I also know something else: That your *different* neurochemistry alone isn't enough to make you very sick. You were well until you were 13. Something must have caused an imbalance of neurotransmitters at that age so severe that it made you want to end your life. What if we were to systematically search for those other things that caused the neurotransmitter imbalance and made you so sick? What if we found them and took care of them, one by one? What if your blood cells returned to normal and flowed freely in the brain? What if we dissolved those microclots in your blood so they don't clog up your brain capillaries anymore? What if we normalized your sugar dysregulation? What if we regulated your hormones better? Do you think things could change?"

As Debbie listened intently, I took the opportunity to broach the next crucial subject. I told her that right then it was extremely dangerous for her not to take Prozac and that she needed her antidepressant medication desperately. I further added that I would do my best to help her get off Prozac eventually. I told her I had succeeded in that with many other patients—not all, but many. Finally, I asked her if she would do me a great favor and agree to take Prozac.

Then it happened. She said she would take Prozac. Her mother, who had watched the whole proceeding with rapt attention, nearly fell off her chair. "What did you say, Debbie?" she blurted. I told the mother that Debbie had agreed to take Prozac. She asked her daughter directly if what she heard indeed was what Debbie had said. Debbie nodded her head. I was certain I saw a faint smile on Debbie's face.

"Injured tissues don't lie, do they?" Choua asked when I finished telling him about Debbie's visit.
"I guess not," I replied.
"So what was that miracle about?"
"Miracle? What miracle?"
"You missed the miracle, didn't you?" he asked, then winked. "That, Mr. Pathologist, was the miracle of observation. Don't you remember what you wrote in *What Do Lions Know About Stress?*
"What?"
"When one knows something, one cannot *unknow* it. A single drop of Debbie's blood told her more than you or her other doctors could have. And that, sir, was the *miracle of observation.*" Choua laughed out loud.
"Yes sir, Mr. Choua Know-It-All!" I replied caustically.

THE MIRACLE OF KNOWLEDGE

"This month you also saw Dirk. Tell me about him," Choua went on.

"You're a scamp." I couldn't suppress a smile. "Is this diatribe going to end sometime?"

"Go on, tell me about that young man," he prodded.

"He saw me for chronic fatigue syndrome, persistent muscle pains of fibromyalgia, disabling brain fog, and depression. He did surprisingly well. He looks well rested, but still suffers from bouts of depression. During the last visit, he said his depression wasn't so bad. He's learning to pull himself up when he begins to sink into depression."

"That's nice. How does he do it?"

"I asked him about that. He read some of my books and tried some autoregulation methods."

"What helped him most?"

"I asked him if he knew which components of our integrative program gave him the most benefit. 'I think everything helped,' he replied. 'Your protein and peptides protocols helped, and so did the vitamins, minerals, essential oils, and herbal protocols. I don't think it was any one thing. Allergy treatment benefited me and autoregulation helped."

Dirk had made some gracious remarks about how some of my writings had helped him recognize the nature of his suffering and learn to cope with his afflictions. Next, he told me what he had omitted when I first saw him six months earlier. Dirk is a gifted painter. During the late 1980s, his work was exhibited at some New York galleries and drew much critical acclaim. After he became sick in 1989, he was unable to finish any paintings. He would paint, get disgusted, and destroy his canvas. He finished with a gentle smile, saying, "But, incredibly, I finished three paintings in the last two weeks that I consider some of my best work." He talked some more.

"What do you think of Dirk's case history?" Choua's words brought me back.

"Very inspiring! I told you so."

"Is that a supernatural event? A case of anecdotal spontaneous recovery? Or a miracle?" Choua asked, his face beaming with satisfaction.

"I choose to call it a miracle," I replied, going along with the gag.

HEALING: THE MIRACLE OF A MIRACLE

"What happens when a seriously ill patient realizes the *limits* of his physician's understanding of the healing phenomena?" Choua asked.

"He begins to look for hope and healing elsewhere," I answered.

"Quite right! Quite right!" Choua spoke excitedly. "He begins to see what healing really is: a miracle in the profoundest sense of the word. What else does he do?"

"He recognizes that there isn't much point in his accepting his physician's prognosis," I guessed.

"How can he? He cannot *unknow* what he knows. Once a patient recognizes deficiencies in his doctor's knowledge of his illness, how can he continue to blindly accept the doctor as the oracle? The patient then learns to trust his higher being. He begins to believe in *Someone* who can make a difference—and that's the beginning of his hope for a miracle. It happened with James, and with David, and the woman with brain cancer. And thousands of your other patients. And millions of other Debbies and Dirks in other doctors' offices. It happens every day, though patients often don't share their insights into healing with their mainstream doctors very often."

"Why?" I asked.

"Because they know their doctors won't believe them. They don't wish to offend their doctors, nor do they wish their doctors to poke fun at what their inward eyes discern. Don't you see miracles dying in doctors' offices every day?"

DYING OF A CANCER IMPLANTED IN THE HEAD

Some weeks ago, a woman in her early sixties consulted me for follow-up care for a colon cancer that had been removed about three years earlier. She knew me previously as a pathologist, because my name appeared on her colon biopsy report as well as on the final pathology report prepared for her excised cancer. Her cancer had spread to the regional lymph nodes, but there had been no evidence of a spread of cancer to other body organs. Three years later, she consulted me as a practitioner of integrative medicine. I reviewed the reports of her recent blood tests and scans and was relieved to find no demonstrable evidence of a recurrent tumor in the colon or metastasis elsewhere in the body. I also learned from her that her brother had died of colon cancer and so did her uncle.

She looked frightened and spoke repeatedly about her urgency to sell her house and attend to some other personal business matters. Given her reassuring recent medical records, I couldn't understand why she was so distraught. Toward the end of my consultation, I asked her if there were other health issues that she hadn't yet told me about.

She became agitated and replied, "Dr. Ali, my oncologist told me I might have five years after I finish chemotherapy. That was three years ago. When I wake up in the morning, I think of the remaining two years. On some days, I actually count the days I have left."

Her words shocked me, but I recovered quickly. Slowly and as gently as I could, I went over her recent blood test results and scans a second time and tried to reassure her that those records didn't reveal any signs of cancer. In the end I could tell she wasn't convinced.

"She's dying of cancer all right," Choua spoke as he followed me out of the room.
"Dying of cancer?" I stopped cold, stunned by Choua's comment. "Did you see something in her records I missed?"
"No, she has no demonstrable cancer," he replied.
"Then why did you say she is dying of cancer?" I asked, annoyed.
"She's not dying of a recurrent colon cancer she doesn't have. She's dying of the cancer her oncologist planted in her head," he replied curtly and fell silent.

I looked at him. His face suddenly turned blank. He seemed to have traveled a million miles in that moment. I knew I had lost him. It was as if he was suddenly called away from me and was then utterly oblivious of the physical reality around him. Such lapses in his attention are not unusual, but he usually returns to the subject after several minutes. I waited for him to return. My thoughts wandered and settled on a passage on hope and healing I had written for *Canary*. Below, I include that passage:

HOPE AND HEALING

Hope *is* healing. Hope is life. Indeed, the human life span is incompatible with the true absence of hope. Absence of hope is *the* most difficult problem I face when I see patients who have suffered from severe, paralyzing fatigue. They have usually undergone extensive diagnostic testing and received multiple drug therapies before I see them. Hopes were dashed as each new set of drug therapies left them weaker and sicker. Thus, my first task is to create hope, and the second is to sustain it. I prepare my patients for recovery by explaining that the therapy may take several weeks, sometimes several months.

When is hope false? When is it true? When is holding out hope for someone inappropriate? When is it pure deception?

Dr. Ali, Billy was such a stunningly beautiful baby no one could look at him only once. Then he grew into a strong six-feet-two young man. His grades in high school were so good. When we drove him to MIT, my husband and I thought we were the luckiest people in the world. And now this! I see him struggle, going from one room to another. He used to weigh 168. When he came down with this thing—whatever it is—he went down to 148. God knows we saw enough specialists. And they did enough tests and prescribed enough antibiotics and antidepressants. For a while, his weight stayed at 148. Now he is down to 140. No one knows what is eating him from within. He is just melting away, right before his mother's eyes and there is nothing she can do." Bill's mother broke down.

I sat motionless, looking at a Monet print hung on the office wall, not wanting to look into Bill's or his mother's eyes. I had no ready answers for either of them. Did I see absence of hope for Bill? No! Did I think I could tell them about it flatly? No. Can hope be dispensed from a prescription pad for every chronic fatiguer? Is every patient ready for the firm assertions that I make in this book about chronic fatigue? There are times when all a physician can do for a patient is to grieve with him.

After a while I looked at them. Bill and his mom were studying my face with intense eyes. "You will get better." I forced a smile and started asking some questions.

HOPE MYOPIA

Hope is *never* false in medicine—provided we have the courage to dismiss the proclamations of drug medicine when its tools fail. Hope is never false if we accept the enduring truth that every form of suffering carries with it a possibility for some spiritual search and rewards — an opportunity for enlightenment. Enlightenment, Jean Paul Sartre wrote, begins on the other side of despair.

Hope myopia—a lack of hope based on a lack of understanding of the true nature of the healing process—is pervasive among the disease doctors of drug medicine. Physicians are trained to look for quick responses from their drugs and scalpels. Such strategies work well when problems we confront are acute and life-threatening but fail utterly when we have to deal with slow, insidious degenerative and immune disorders. The disease doctors of drug medicine are incarcerated in mental boxes of their own making. The fact is that serious environmental, nutritional, degenerative, and immune disorders can be managed—and their recurrences prevented—only through focus on nutrition, environment, self-regulation and spiritual search. Chronic viral syndromes also fall in the same general category. Unfortunately, such an approach has come to be regarded as quackery by mainstream medicine in the United States.

SIMPLE TRUTHS
AND COMPLICATED LIES

Chronic fatigue syndrome reflects a complex interaction between cerebral dysfunction, trigger factors, and social attitudes, and is complicated by secondary symptoms. There will be no simple explanation.

British Medical Journal 306:1558; 1993.

The *Journal* does not see any hope for understanding the fatigue problem. I do.

The public will believe a simple lie in preference to a complicated truth, de Tocqueville wrote in his commentary on early Americans. If de Tocqueville were to return and visit our chronic fatigue centers today, he would find the opposite: Our fatigue experts prefer complicated lies to simple truths.

The story of chronic fatigue syndrome has become a web of complicated lies, and our fatigue experts continue to weave new yarns every day. On a positive note, chronic fatiguers are beginning to see the simple truth. Here is how a patient put it to me recently:

Dr. Ali, it took me a long time to finally understand what you have been trying to explain to me. I know now that only I can pull myself out of this problem. You can only guide me. Of course, IV drips and immunotherapy shots and auto-reg do their part.

Chronic fatigue states are reversible. We need to suspend our disbelief of the enormous restorative potential of nutritional, environmental, and self-regulatory methods and simply try them.

HOPE AND DISEASE DOCTORS OF DRUG MEDICINE

How can a rheumatologist instill hope for a cure in a patient with rheumatoid arthritis? After all, he knows that his steroids only further suppress an injured immune system, and gold injections, as useful as they may be in reducing symptoms, never cure rheumatoid arthritis.

How can a gastroenterologist create hope for a patient with ulcerative colitis? He knows his steroids suppress the immune system and his Azulfidine never cures ulcerative colitis.

How can a dermatologist ever bring hope to a patient with eczema? He knows his steroids suppress the immune system and his skin creams only hide the underlying problem.

How can a pulmonologist create hope for a cure for a patient with asthma? He knows his steroids suppress the immune system, and his bronchodilator drugs cannot normalize the underlying molecular abnormalities.

How can a cardiologist create hope for a cure for his patients with coronary heart disease? He is absolutely convinced the heart disease of his patient is completely irreversible.

There are yet other reasons why hope myopia continues to flourish among the practitioners of N^2D^2 medicine (see Glossary). There are lawyers who advise physicians against hope—it is the fabric that lawsuits are made of, they assert. There are insurance companies that advise against hope—'promise nothing so you may be sued for nothing,' they say in words that cannot be heard, only inferred. The editors of our medical journals do their part—'what's not double-blinded and crossed-over is not to be trusted,' they admonish. Hope, of course, can neither be blinded nor crossed-over. There is even a new genre of quality assurance personnel in our hospitals — brainwashed by the gurus of *total quality management* (TQM) at the Joint Commission on Accreditation of Healthcare Organizations — who believe that what cannot be *quantified* cannot be *real*. Thus, hope, being unquantifiable, is of no interest to them.

Is it hard, then, to understand why disease doctors of drug medicine do not like the subject of hope in medicine? Why would they?

Can every chronic fatiguer wholly regain his full energy level? If not recovery, what percentage *can* he recover? How shall we compute the percentage by which we must reduce hope for him? How do we measure the "quantity" of hope? Who should decide that? The editor of some prestigious journal? Someone sitting on a state licensing board? A medical ethicist? Should it be a lawyer? Or perhaps a judge?

Some years ago, I heard a physician vehemently petition a group of physicians to have the hospital seek a court order allowing him to operate on his patient. The woman in question — a bag lady hospitalized for a large abscess around her rectum that caused a blockage — had steadfastly fought all attempts by her surgeons to persuade her to sign a surgical consent. The principal argument of the physician was that the patient was most assuredly going to die if this operation was delayed for too long and that she clearly was not intelligent enough to understand the risks she faced. Some days later, I ran into the physician and asked him about the woman with the rectal abscess. "Her abscess burst into her rectum, she passed out all the junk in her stool, and signed out against medical advice." He shrugged his shoulders and walked away. So much for dragging courts into medical issues!

CLINICAL BENEFITS OF HOPELESSNESS

Late in the evening of the day Choua and I talked about science, medicine and miracles, I saw two older physicians, a man and a woman, on TV discuss terminal care for patients with cancer. They spoke about how hard it was for them to decide when a patient becomes terminal—and how much harder it was to communicate that determination to the patient and his family. What seemed to concern them most was their eagerness to help the patient put his house in order. There were the usual concerns about the patients completing their wills and making other arrangements for their deaths. There was also much talk about the need for the dying person to make peace with family members and resolve long-festering conflicts. I had heard such discussions hundreds of times at cancer meetings.

"Who decides when a patient is terminal?" Choua asked when the program came to a close.

"Doctors, of course. When the cancer is spread beyond any reasonable hope of control, it isn't too difficult to see that a patient is terminal."

"It isn't too difficult to play God. Is that it?" he frowned.

"Someone has to," I replied, irritated. "If physicians can't, who can? Some hospital administrator? A lawyer? Or a judge?"

"Why does anyone have to make such a decision?"

"Get real, Choua," I replied with growing irritation. "Somebody has to."

"Why?" he pressed.

"For one thing, the family usually insists on knowing how long their loved one will live."

"Do you *have* to tell a person he's terminal just because his *family* insists you do?" he asked testily, then added, "That's pretty dumb, isn't it?"

"I didn't mean it that way," I protested.

"What *did* you mean?" he groused.

"Dying persons need to make preparations, don't they?" I asked, annoyed.

"Did you ever ask anyone you *believed to be terminal* if he preferred to be told that he was dying?"

"You distort everything," I scolded him. "Caring for a dying person is a serious business. That's not a time for logic or debate."

"Is it a time to be illogical?" he asked contemptuously.

"Get off my case, will you?" I pleaded.

"There's a profound irony there." Choua's voice suddenly fell into a whisper. "Doctors foolishly attribute to themselves powers that are clearly divine. They're distressed to have to make decisions that do not need to be made."

"That's ludicrous. People need to..."

"No one *needs* to be told he is dying," Choua cut me off sharply.

"That's absurd," I snapped back. "There are times when there is no hope for life."

"No hope!" he scowled. "Tell me, what are the clinical benefits of hopelessness for the patient?"

"What?" I was stumped by his question. "Clinical benefits of hopelessness?"

"Yes! What are the clinical benefits of hopelessness for a patient?" he repeated his question.

"Oh God! You're impossible today," I reprimanded. "There are no clinical benefits of hopelessness for anyone."

"Then why create hopelessness for any patient?" he asked tersely.

Why create hopelessness for a patient? I muttered under my breath. Choua had asked a question that never crossed my mind. Of course, no one in his right mind would ever think of deliberately creating hopelessness for a sick person. I had attended hundreds of medical conferences in which the participants engaged in scholarly dissertations of scientific, ethical and moral issues involved in determining the terminal status of a patient. Then they struggled to decide how to communicate that information to the dying person. Such discussions were always somber. And now there was Choua belittling the issue while poking fun at the whole world of oncology.

I tried to recall if anyone had ever looked at the problem the way Choua did. If there are no clinical benefits of hopelessness, why create it for anyone, regardless of how certain a physician might be of his patient's impending death? He had raised a troubling question, and I didn't quite know how to settle it in my own mind.

I felt Choua's stare on my face and began, "What do you suppose a physician should do when he really thinks the patient is terminal?"

"Have you ever determined anyone's *terminality?*"

"What is terminality?" I teased.

"You know what I mean," he said curtly. "Have you ever told a patient he is terminal?" he asked back.

"No."

"Why not?"

"I suppose I never considered it necessary."

"Never considered it *necessary?*" he shot back. "If you don't ever consider it necessary, why do you think oncologists do?"

"I don't know, Choua. I never thought about it. Why don't you answer your own question?" I asked.

"Because you holistic physicians are different."

"How so?"

"Because you don't play God. You see your role in that whole scenario clearly."

"And, what, pray tell me, is our role in such a scenario?" I asked sarcastically.

"To do what you can and not play the Divine," he replied with a wink.

"How do you know oncologists don't consider that their role as well?"

"If that were so, why would those oncologists on TV make

such a fuss about how to determine who is terminal?"

"They weren't making a fuss," I rebuked him.

"You missed the whole point," Choua chuckled.

"What's the point?" I asked, exasperated.

"Holistic physicians like you are different from oncologists. That's the point. You prescribe natural remedies. You administer nutrient and herbal injections and IV drips. You infuse ozone and hydrogen peroxide. All those therapies enhance a patient's own defenses. And you talk about the healing energy of the divine *presence* that surrounds and permeates each of us. You don't realize that when you do that, there is no reason for you to pronounce anyone terminal. You don't see how deftly you sidestep the whole mess—or, should I say, *someone* does the sidestepping for you."

"What mess? And who sidesteps that *for* me?" I asked, baffled.

A mystical smile spread on Choua's face as he turned and looked out the window. What mess? I wondered. And who does the sidestepping for me? Several moments passed. Then I began to see what Choua meant. He was right. I had never consciously made the decision not to discuss the terminal status of a patient. It never seemed relevant to me. I simply did what seemed right for each individual patient. Now that Choua brought the subject up, I began to see that the decision had been made for me by someone else. Who? Of course, who else? I looked at Choua. He seemed lost in the distant horizon. *Clinical benefits of hopelessness*, Choua's words returned and took on new meanings. Is life possible without hope? The question took shape in my mind. Not for too long, came the reply. Why should a physician pronounce any patient dead before his time? To help a patient draw his last will? Now if that isn't the dumbest reason of all for condemning a person with a declaration of death. Choua had fired a lot of questions at me. Now the answers began to take shape in my mind.

"It's different with oncologists." Choua's words brought me back.

"How so?"

"When an oncologist administers chemo to a patient he considers terminal, he's torn inside by the knowledge of what his drugs are going to do to the sick person."

"As usual, you exaggerate. Oncologists use toxic chemo drugs in the hope that they can cure or control cancer."

"Is that really true?" he scowled. "Is that what you and other pathologists see at autopsies? Don't you think they read their oncology journals and know the statistics? Even with all the distortions, chemo statistics for curing and controlling cancer stink."

"Sometimes they do succeed and..."

"Succeed in what?" he rudely cut me off. "Chemo drugs are poisons that suck out whatever life is left in ill persons. Debilitated by their tumors, weakened by pain and suffering, the poor patients are ill-equipped to withstand the medical pronouncements of their doctors. They can ill afford the punishment of chemo. They become nauseated and can't eat anything. They develop ulcers in their mouths and guts. Their pain becomes more intense, and they begin to lose hope. Oncologists know all that better than anyone else—and they're torn by that knowledge. Still, they're expected to do something. Their great gurus of chemo have admonished them to shun holistic physicians and their nutrient and herbal therapies. Oncologists can't use their poisons. And they can't use supportive nutrient and herbal remedies. They are not permitted to believe in miracles—the chemo gurus have also warned them against the anecdotal spontaneous cures of cancer. The oncologists desperately need a way out, and the idea of terminality comes handy. Pronouncement of terminal status absolves the oncologists of all guilt and conflict. It is a neat solution to a messy problem." Choua finished with a frown.

"So you're saying that oncologists just let people die. What a ghastly thing to say! You're a master of distortion, Choua. You're..."

"It's different with holistic physicians," he calmly cut me off.

"How?" I asked, exasperated.

"When a holistic physician ministers to the critically ill, he is sustained by the fact that all his work is supportive—if his therapies won't help, they most assuredly will not hurt. So deep in the core of his heart, he hopes and prays for a miracle. And, of course, sometimes he does witness miracles. The holistic physician has no urgency to declare his patient terminal and unfit for poisonous chemo, as an oncologist does. The holistic..."

"Oh, c'mon Choua," I interrupted him. "You can't help but distort the truth. You..."

"Don't you see something that simple?" He didn't let me finish my sentence. "Declaration of terminality of a patient suits the oncologist. The oncologist can then safely—and without remorse—send the patient to some hospice to die. That's the clinical benefit of hopelessness. Except sometimes there are problems with that too."

"What?"

"Do you remember what Donald told you?"

"Donald who?"

"The fellow who gives music therapy in a New York City hospice."

"What did he say?"

"He said there are three types of patients in his hospice: Those who die fast, those who die slowly, and those who refuse to die. There is a problem with the third group. The hospice administrators do not know what to do with them. Have you ever thought how difficult that might be for them? When you and your colleagues meet to review the clinical progress of your patients, you try to figure out ways of moving your patients along faster. What can the hospice doctors and administrators do? I mean, they can't undertake some project to expedite the death of those who refuse to die, can they?"

"You're nuts!" I nearly screamed at him. "Your warped mind endlessly spins tales of horror. Only this time you have gone too far."

"Don't you see?" Choua went on evenly. "The clinical benefits of hopelessness..."

"You're being mean and vicious," I shouted angrily, unable to control my frustration. "What oncologists do is prepare the patient and his family for death. Don't you see that the dying have some business to transact before they pass away? Choua, I know you don't live in the real world. You don't care for the seriously sick. But there are such things as wills and business matters that must be attended to. Then there are other more compelling unresolved personal and family issues. A person with an advanced cancer must be told that. And..."

"Nonsense!" he erupted. "A person with an advanced cancer does not need to be told that he has advanced cancer. He already *knows* that. Can you recall a single very sick patient who *you* thought may not make it who needed to be told by *you* that he was very sick? The seriously ill have their own visceral-intuitive sense of their inner state. They know better than you what needs to be done. Remember, they *live in* the body every moment that you doctors examine only once a week or once a month. They *know!*"

"Are you saying oncologists should never tell patients the truth about their illness?" I refused to yield, even though I understood and agreed with Choua's argument. "Do you have any idea what havoc that would create?"

"The truth?" he groused contemptuously. "You don't get it, Mr. Pathologist, do you? Who gave you the monopoly on truth? Have you never seen a hospitalized patient whose chart was littered with 'Don't resuscitate' orders and yet he defied all the prognostications by his doctors and walked out of the hospital?"

"Yes, I have," I confessed meekly, then added, "But those are miracles."

"Precisely! Precisely!" Choua grinned broadly.

"But the miracles don't happen often," I persisted.

"That's not the point. As long as there is a one in 1,000 chance that a patient can recover—by a miracle, if you wish to call it that—no one has the right to deny him that possibility. Don't you see something that simple?" he goaded.

"Choua, you aren't a clinician. You're a mere theorist. You don't treat patients and certainly you have no concept of what it means to lose a patient after you've worked day and night for that patient as oncologists do. You sit on your high horse pontificating. What do you know about an oncologist's anguish anyway? Your insensitivity is appalling—and it is embarrassing," I scolded him.

Choua stiffened, looked at me with blank eyes for several moments, then lowered his head. We were silent for some time.

I HAVE TO GO POISON SOMEONE

"Yeah, it's tough for oncologists," he broke the silence in a soft tone. "I don't doubt that."

"Most oncologists I know are caring, compassionate

physicians who try to do their best with the tools they have against those dreaded malignant diseases," I said in a conciliatory tone as well, then added, "It's not their fault that their chemo drugs sometimes don't work."

"Not sometimes," he countered. "Say, they rarely work. How many autopsies have you performed on patients who were *cured* by their oncologists?"

"Oh, God! You don't ever relent, do you?" I felt my anger returning.

"How often have you heard an oncologist tell you 'I have to go poison someone'?" he asked gently.

I suppressed a smile. He had deftly defused my anger. He knew that was exactly the sentence many oncologists had spoken to me over the years when they left my office after reviewing the microscopic slides of their patients' cancers. It is hard to stay angry with him on such occasions. Rogue! I muttered under my breath and decided not to answer his question.

"The declaration of terminality of a patient suits the patient's oncologist," Choua went on.

"What an awful thing to say!" I scolded him again.

"What are the clinical benefits of hopelessness?" Choua repeated.

This time Choua's words returned to amuse me. He does have a way of making things funny, I thought to myself. Who else could find clinical benefits in hopelessness? Chemo drugs are potent cellular poisons, of that there is no doubt. Nutrient and herbal drips may not help some patients with advanced cancers to any measurable degrees, but they do not hurt. There could be no doubt about that either. I couldn't disagree with what Choua said. It's just that the words he chooses to state his case are offensive to me. How would an oncologist take that? I wondered.

THE CHOICE:
DIE LIVING OR LIVE DYING

"You are terminal, aren't you?" Choua asked after a while with a twinkle.

"What?" I asked, taken by sudden inquiry.

"You're terminal. I'm terminal," he winked again, then added, "The miracle is that every day we live."

"In that sense everyone is terminal," I said, recovering and laughing.

"Tell me in what sense are you *not* terminal?" he asked, turning solemn.

"Get off my case, will you?" I rebuked him.

"Since everyone is terminal, a physician has but one choice."

"Pray, tell me," I said sarcastically.

"He can help people die living or he can condemn them to live dying."

"What was that?" I asked, confused by his play on words. "Say that again, Choua."

Choua turned on his heels and, without waiting for me to finish my sentence, walked out of the room. Choua often argues his case passionately—and nowhere is he more passionate than when he assaults what he considers pseudoscience and medical deceptions. Sometimes I deliberately provoke him. Sometimes he needles me. On that day he had been especially hard on oncologists. What are the clinical benefits of hopelessness?

Choua's words returned. I found that concept an interesting way to look at what I know is one of the most difficult areas in the care of patients with advanced cancer. Then my thoughts drifted to his words about what the open eye of the scientist sees and what the unopened eye of a mystic discerns. What was that all about? I wondered. I had wanted him to explain himself on that matter, but he jumped subjects so fast that I forgot all about it until after he was gone. What is it that the open eye of a scientist cannot see but the closed eye of a mystic can? What did he mean? I decided to take up that subject when I saw him next.

WHAT THE OPEN EYE CANNOT SEE

Choua visited us at home a few days later. I stood by the window, looking at the Hudson River. I remembered his comments about the scientist and the mystic and broached the subject.

"We talked about a lot of things the other day, Choua. You said something about a mystic's closed eye discerning things that a scientist's open eye can't see. What was that all about?"

"I meant what I said," he replied with a smile.

"Can you elaborate? I mean, can you say that in words that a mortal like myself can understand?" I mocked.

"Science is the conquered terrain of the mystic," he replied, ignoring my sarcasm. "A mystic's unopened eye usually discerns what the open eye of the scientist sees centuries, sometimes millennia, later."

"Wow! That's some statement. Can you give me a specific example of something that mystics saw and *described* centuries before scientists did?"

"A specific example?" his forehead furrowed.

"Yes, something concrete that a sinner like me can comprehend," I goaded.

Choua looked at me, then out the window. Moments later, he backed off from the window, then turned to scan piles of books on end tables by the sofa and others on the floor. Not finding any book to his liking, he ambled to my library. Moments later, he returned holding an opened book in his hand and spoke, "This is *Three Ways of Asian Wisdom* by Nancy Wilson Ross published by Simon and Schuster. Listen, I'll read you a passage on page 65:

The sun never sets or rises. When people think the sun is setting, he [the sun] only changes about after reaching the end of the day and makes night below and day to what is on the other side. Then, when people think he rises in the morning, he only shifts himself about after reaching the end of the night, and makes day below and night to what is on the other side. In truth, he does not set at all.

Ross is quoting from a section of the Veda known as Brahmanas. Now, tell me, how old are the Veda?" Choua asked as he looked up from the page of *Three Ways of Asian Wisdom.*

"Astounding!" I couldn't help myself.

"Take a guess. How many thousands of years was that passage written before Copernicus challenged the Ptolemaic view that the sun revolves around the earth?"

"Three thousand years? Maybe more."

"What happened to Copernicus?"

"He was rejected and ridiculed."

"By whom?"

"By the scientists of his time." The words slipped from my mouth.

"How many thousands of years were the Veda written before Galileo Galilei's time?"

"Galileo was born in 1564, twenty-one years after Copernicus died."

"What did they do to Galileo when he said that the sun doesn't go around the earth but that the earth goes around the sun?"

"You know the answer. He was incarcerated in his home and forced to recant his scientific observations on pain of death."

"What the open eye cannot see," he murmured softly and left the room.

I have been privileged to witness many miracles. I close this chapter with a miracle I described in *The Canary and Chronic Fatigue*.

DR. ALI, YOUR SWORD STORY DID IT

Andrew had been disabled with chronic fatigue for about a year when he first consulted me. I sensed something different about him within moments of his entering my office. I finished scanning the chronic fatigue questionnaire I use in my practice and looked up to ask him some questions about his health. He stared at me with sad eyes. As I asked questions regarding his medical problems, he kept interrupting his answers to talk about his two daughters who apparently suffered from many of the symptoms he described. Finally, I said, "Your daughters are not here. You are. Once you get better, we can take care of your daughters."

"No, you won't," Andrew blurted.

"Okay, then, we won't." His answer took me by surprise, but I recovered quickly. "Let's talk about you."

"You can't help my daughters, Doc," Andrew spoke softly this time.

"Fine! Fine! Tell me when did you..."

"You can't help my daughters because my wife won't let you," he interrupted me.

"Let's just talk about you, Andrew," I said with some frustration.

"Doc, I wish you could help my daughters, but you can't because my wife thinks your work is hocus-pocus." Andrew became sad, then sat up quickly. "My wife is a successful businesswoman. And she is a very strong woman. I have been disabled with this thing and can't do anything for my daughters. They are sick every month, and I see their pediatrician prescribe antibiotics every month, just the way my pediatrician did for me. I'm very afraid for them."

I saw Andrew ten weeks later for a follow-up visit. There was no sign of any improvement. I saw my notation, "concerned about two daughters," in his chart and wondered how the situation at home might be. I decided not to ask him any questions about that.

Andrew continued to receive immunotherapy from our office, but did not keep his appointment for a follow-up visit with me until several months later. Then he came in one day, his face joyful. I wondered if the situation with his daughters had changed, but said nothing. Next, I started to make entries in the chronic fatigue outcome sheet that I use in my practice for research studies.

"Tell me, Andrew, how is your energy level these days?" I asked.
"Excellent!" he beamed.
"Excellent?" I asked in disbelief.
"Excellent. I'm running a marathon," he crowed.
"Running a marathon?" I was stunned.
"Yup! I'm running a marathon." Andrew became serious.

Chronic fatigue patients do not run marathons — not those who have been disabled for months. I was not prepared for this. Without being too obvious, I thumbed through the chart to see if I had the right chart, to ensure he was the patient I thought he was, the father of two daughters. "Concerned about two daughters," I saw my notation in the chart and knew there was no mistake there.

"I'm not sure that's a good idea, Andrew," I began. "Marathons shouldn't be run by people who are just coming out of chronic fatigue," I counseled.
"I knew that's what you would say, Doc. But I am not coming out of chronic fatigue now. I have been out of chronic fatigue. I waited for three months before I decided to come and tell you about it. Your story did it. Yup, your story did it for me." Andrew grinned broadly.

I tell a lot of stories to my patients to help them understand the nature of this beast, chronic fatigue, and to help them cope with their unique brand of suffering. What story was Andrew talking about? I wondered. I looked up. Andrew was studying my face with his intense blue eyes.

"Dr, Ali, your sword story did it. You remember your sword story, Doc, don't you?" Andrew flashed a smile.

I often tell my patients the sword story to make some points about the spiritual search and its rewards. It goes something like this:

There was a ferocious captain in Genghis Khan's army during the invasion of India. He killed people with his sword at the least provocation and often without any provocation at all. His reputation preceded him wherever he went. On this occasion, after he entered a town, he thunderously demanded from his lieutenants to know if anyone was left alive.

"No one, sir! No one except for this spiritual man," a lieutenant answered.
"Aha! A spiritual fool!" he thundered. "Take me to the fool," he ordered.

His lieutenant led him to an ancient small temple with a broken wooden door. The captain ordered the door smashed down. Within moments, his lieutenants smashed the door down. The captain entered the tiny courtyard. A thin man in a loincloth and wooden sandals stood still in the middle of the courtyard. The captain contemptuously looked at the spiritual man and roared,

"Do you know who I am?"
"No, I don't," the spiritual man answered meekly.
"You don't know who I am?" the captain asked, shaking with rage.
"No, I don't," the spiritual man repeated his words timidly.

The captain pulled his sword from its sheath and flashed it with his full might. "I can slice through your body and not blink an eye," he thundered again.

Everyone standing behind the captain froze, their eyes fixed on the spiritual man. Time seemed to stop. The spiritual man stood silently, looking back at the captain with vacant eyes. Then he asked in a whisper, "Do you know who I am, sir?"

"Who are you?" the captain roared again, thrusting his sword forward until it nearly touched the spiritual man's abdomen.

"I could have your sword slice through me and not blink an eye," the spiritual man answered.

The captain trembled in his feet and walked out without saying a word.

"How did the sword story help you?" I asked Andrew in good humor.

"Your sword story did it, Doc. I'm serious," Andrew began with a grin. "A few months after I saw you last, my wife took a lover and threw me out. Suddenly, there I was. I had no wife. No home. No job. And I couldn't see my daughters. What would I tell my daughters anyway? I had nothing left. There was no reason for me to go on. No reason to fight back at all. No reason to live. There was nothing there. Just darkness. Then into that darkness came the sword and the man in the loincloth and wooden sandals. Then I don't quite know what happened — except that I wasn't afraid anymore. Nothing mattered anymore. I wasn't afraid. I think that did it! I wasn't afraid anymore. I guess I was just like that spiritual man. I thought I could have anyone slice through me and I wouldn't blink an eye — just like the man in the loincloth and wooden sandal. I began to move around and then I found the energy to start walking and then running. Before I knew it, I was preparing for the marathon. This is how it all happened. I was free at last — free of fear and free of anger. I wasn't a victim anymore. I knew there was something out there. I didn't know what, but *it* was out there, and it didn't seem to matter that I couldn't know *it* any better. I wasn't tired anymore. Honest Doc, that's what happened." Andrew shook his head warmly. There was nothing for me to say.

The story came back to me some weeks after I saw Andrew. In a flash, I saw him the way he looked during the first visit — distraught, deeply hurt, interrupting his answers about his health to talk about his daughters. Then I saw clearly what I had failed to see then: He was going through a profound change—a spiritual change, through his suffering for his daughters. He didn't see it then, nor did I. Now I know it was not the sword story that did it. It was his love for his daughters that did it. He suffered for his daughters and, through that suffering, he came to the truth — that there is something, *someone,* beyond our bodily senses and beyond all reach of the intellect that can sustain us when nothing else does. He went to that third dimension — the spiritual — that none of us is destined to know, and returned with a change, a transformation that neither he nor I could have known with our bodily senses nor with our clever thinking. The spiritual man in the loincloth and wooden sandals in the sword story was just a little spark that he saw during his journey.

ABSTRACT

Improved Myocardial Perfusion
with EDTA Chelation Therapy

Majid Ali, MD; Omar Ali, MD; Alfred Fayemi, MD;
Judy Juco, MD; Carol Grieder, RN

Presented at the American Academy of Preventive Medicine, 1995)

Efficacy of EDTA chelation therapy for reversing coronary artery disease was evaluated with clinical outcome and thallium myocardial perfusion studies in 26 patients (21 males; 5 females). The mean age was 65 years (range: 42-76). Duration of therapy was 1.5 years (range: 5 months-9 years). Scoring system for clinical outcome was as follows: Excellent, 100% reduction of symptoms and drug dosage; good, 75% symptom and drug dose reduction; moderate, 25% to 50% symptom and drug dose reduction; and poor, less than 25% symptom and drug dose reduction.

Clinical outcome data are as follows: excellent 61%, good 17%, moderate 13%, and poor 9%. Pre- and post-chelation myocardial perfusion scans were available for comparison study in six patients. Objective evidence of significant improvement in perfusion was observed in five of six patients (scan to be presented). A careful review of the records of two patients showed that angioplasty was performed unnecessarily when coronary vasospasm was misdiagnosed as coronary artery occlusion.

The above study was presented at the 1995 annual meeting

of the American Academy of Preventive Medicine in New York. The full details of that study were subsequently published in *The Journal of Integrative Medicine*, 1:37; 1997.

My colleagues are now collating data for a larger study with a longer period of follow-up for publication. So far, the clinical outcome data for that more extensive study are just as encouraging as in the study cited above.

****

You sometimes speak of gravity as essential and inherent to matter. Pray, do not ascribe this notion to me; for the cause of gravity is what I do not pretend to know, and therefore would take more time to consider it.

Isaac Newton

The most beautiful and profound emotion we can experience is the sensation of the mystical. It is the sower of all science...He to whom this emotion is a stranger, who can no longer wonder and stand rapt in awe, is as good as dead.

Albert Einstein

Chapter 2

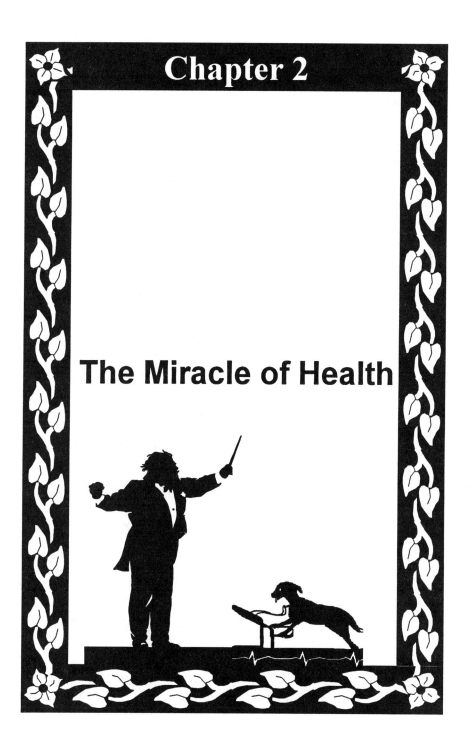

The Miracle of Health

Health is a miracle.

When I was a medical student, what fascinated me most was not how people got sick, but how anyone ever stayed healthy. I thought it was a legitimate question then, and I think it is so now. How much can go wrong in the human body at any time? How much *does* go wrong in the human body at any time? The answer is unimaginable. Consider:

> *Every second that passes, the DNA in each cell of your body is being damaged. Chemical bonds are breaking, DNA strands are snapping, and nucleotide bases are flying off. Each cell loses more than 10,000 bases per day just from spontaneous breakdown of DNA at body temperature. Meanwhile, many cells are dividing and therefore copying DNA, and each copy introduces the possibility of error.*
>
> *Science* 266:1926; 1994

Translation: DNA in each cell in the body has 10,000 chances per day of becoming cancerous, since cancer may be defined as DNA mutation. It has been estimated that there are 100 trillion cells in the human body. Even if this estimate is off by 100 times, and even if the estimate of *Science* is off by another 100 times, it still comes to the possibility of one hundred trillion chances of developing a cancer on any given day. If those are the odds, how does anyone *not* have cancer? If that's not a miracle of health, I don't know what is.

When I study the blood of my patients with a high-resolution microscope, I see some bacteria, yeast and evidence of oxidative damage to plasma proteins and cell membranes of varying degrees in almost all patients. The blood stream of many chronically ill patients is literally a sewer, with dead and dying cells floating everywhere, with bacterial and yeast debris everywhere. I used to wonder why such patients didn't die with multiple infections and abscesses. Now I look at all such conditions as miracles of life.

Other than being an unending miracle, what is health?

What Is Health?

How is health defined in drug medicine? It isn't. The subject of what health is—and what it isn't—is scrupulously avoided in our medical schools, hospitals and physicians' offices. We dismiss any reference to it by mumbling something unintelligible about the physical, mental and emotional aspects of health.

But what are the physical attributes of health? How do we define mental health? What is emotional wholeness? I have attended thousands of medical lectures since entering King Edward Medical College in 1958, yet I can't recall ever hearing a serious attempt to answer these questions. Why?

I never reflected on these questions throughout the more than 25 years that I worked as a disease doctor of drug medicine. It was only when my interest shifted from disease to health that the issue caught my attention. So, what is health?

Health is rising in the morning with a sense of the spiritual—without any need to analyze what the spiritual might be. In health, spirituality—trust in the larger *presence*—displaces the practice of psychology in one's work.

Health, at a deeper level, is resonance with the larger *presence* that permeates and surrounds each of us at all times.

Health is waking up in the morning with a deep sense of gratitude—gratitude not for any particular accomplishment, *but for simply being*. Recently I made some comments about this aspect of health during a lecture at the American Academy of Otolaryngic Allergy. In the audience was a Greek surgeon who later expressed his frustration at my comments, "This is utterly new to my Greek way of thinking." Well, if the concept of gratitude for simply *being* is foreign to us, we need to learn about it.

Health is waking up with a sense of energy, going through a day's work with that same sense of energy and returning to bed at night with it.

Health is having as much energy before meals as after them.

Health is the ability to treasure personal time in silence —alone or with family and friends. Relentless thinking—head fixation, as it may be called—is a major stressor and eventually causes dis-ease and disease.

Health comprises living with dynamic and vigorous bowel ecosystems—having two or three effortless and odorless bowel movements a day without mucus and cramps.

Health comprises dynamic and well-preserved blood, liver and other body ecosystems.

Health is having intact and functioning cell membranes that mark the boundaries between life within the cell and that which exists outside it. The cell membrane separates the internal order of a cell from external disorder. It is a living, breathing, spongy and porous sheet that regulates the two-way energetic-molecular (EM) traffic between cells and the soup of life that bathes them.

Returning to the first element of resonance with the larger *presence*, health is the sum total of all atomic, cellular and molecular resonances that exist within the human frame. I do not consider this an abstract and metaphysical notion. Common sense holds that a part cannot exist without some relationship to the whole. Since each of us is an energy being that is part of the larger world, all of us have a definite relationship with all the energies around us that exist on the planet Earth—and those beyond. It is an elementary fact of physics that all bodies in an energy field resonate with that field. An amoeba resonates just as each cell in the human body does. Such atomic and cellular resonances, in my view, represent the essence of health of a being.

I will illustrate this concept with a simple example. The surface of a healthy cell resonates with a weak negative surface charge of about -3 microvolts. A cancer cell, by contrast, is highly charged and resonates with a much higher charge that may reach a value of -200 to -250 microvolts. In a type of treatment I call tumor potential restoration (TPR), I apply a positive electrode to the surface of a malignant tumor and regularly observe the charge change within seconds—as electrons fly from the center of the tumor toward the surface and then to the electrode with a speed that may exceed thousands of miles per second. Similar energy dynamics, reflecting changes in molecular and cellular resonances, take place in all heathy cells during metabolism and in abnormal cells in other disease states, though we cannot observe them with available technology. I am confident that future advances in physical energy technologies will allow us to observe and document other examples of molecular and cellular resonances.

What is the source of such resonance? We may call it solar radiation, stellar radiation, cosmic or geomagnetic waves, or by any other name. I concede that the core energy aspects of that *presence* are—and I believe, will always remain—unknowable. All the technology of humankind has not explained the essence of those energies—and I believe it never will. No doubt we will learn more about aspects of that *presence* as our technology advances. But my strong sense is that no matter how much our science advances, we will never know the essentially unknowable aspects of that *presence*. Thus, I come full circle back to where I started—that we humans must accept the spiritual as beyond the reach of our physical senses and intellectual capacity.

The concept of the health of cell membranes in my definition of health may seem tedious to some readers. In the following passage, which is an excerpt from the companion volume, *RDA: Rats, Drugs and Assumptions,* I present a conceptual framework for what I call EM medicine.

The essence of EM medicine is to seek a genuine understanding of the energetic-molecular dynamics of cells **before** *the cells are injured, and not on our notions of cellular injury as seen through a microscope after the injury has occurred. All nondrug, restorative therapies that I use to reverse chronic disease, and describe in this series of books, are based on EM dynamics of health. This model of clinical medicine promotes health with natural therapies that revive injured bowel, blood and cellular ecosystems.*

It is not uncommon for me to hear mainstream doctors criticize holistic physicians for their "unscientific" methods. They consider all drug therapies scientific and scornfully dismiss all nondrug, empirical therapies as forms of quackery. The truth is that empiricism in medicine is a valid science. Empirical medicine relies on sound clinical observations—and observation, of course, is the purest of all sciences. Thus, it is far more scientific to base one's restorative therapies on a genuine understanding of bowel, blood and cellular ecosystems than to simply suppress symptoms of disease with drugs. Sick humans are not mere bits of bowel to be examined with a microscope, nor are they slices of diseased skin to be covered with steroid creams. It is far more scientific to consider a sick person as a whole organism in stress and holistically address all the issues of his illness rather than test for one or two hormone levels in the blood and prescribe replacement hormonal therapy.

Drug medicine essentially is the use of drugs that block human energy, detoxification, and digestive-absorptive enzyme systems. Drugs, as useful as they might be in the management of acute illnesses, block normal healing processes—and, hence, do not constitute a true solution to problems caused by damaged body ecosystems. Furthermore, drugs, as we all recognize, eventually lose their effectiveness as human metabolic enzymes devise new ways to bypass their blockade.

WHAT HEALTH IS NOT

Health is not the mere absence of disease. Health has nothing to do with the whimsical notions of RDAs (Recommended Daily Allowances) to prevent a handful of nutrient-deficiency syndromes, nor is it the "balanced diet" prescribed by doctors who practice drug medicine and consider nutritional medicine quackery.

Health is not the euphoria of eating, nor is it the denial of dieting. Health is not preoccupation with recycling past miseries, nor is it pre-cycling feared, future misery. Health is not living with regrets, nor is it an obsession with control in life.

So why do mainstream physicians shun the subject of health? The answer is really quite simple: *None of the essential aspects of health defined in this chapter can be addressed with drugs.* There are no drugs that make us spiritual or bring us gratitude and freedom from anger. There are no drugs that teach us the limbic language of silence or extinguish the oxidative fires of stress. Drugs cannot revive injured energy enzymes, nor can they repair damaged detoxification enzymes. There are no synthetic chemicals that can upregulate energy and fat-burning enzymes. Drugs cannot restore a damaged bowel ecosystem nor can they strengthen a weakened blood ecosystem. Drugs cannot normalize disrupted EM dynamics of the cell and plasma membranes.

Injured tissues heal with nutrients, not with drugs. Indeed, the tools of modern medicine—drugs and surgical scalpels—are singularly ineffective in coping with the stressors of life today and in promoting health.

Food fuels the furnace of metabolism; exercise stokes its fire.

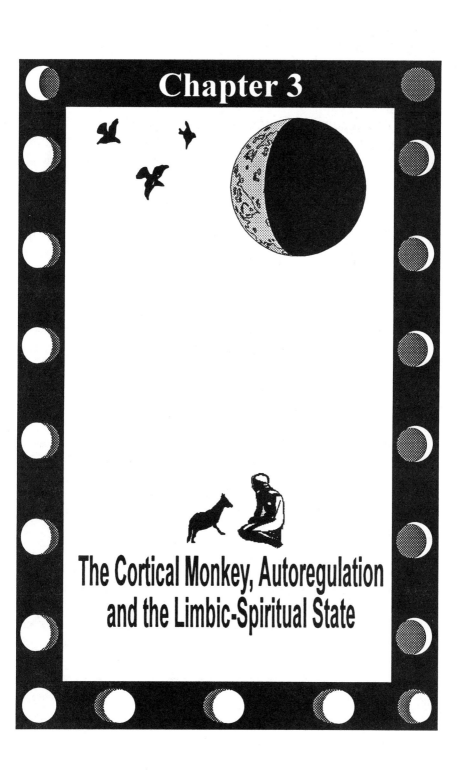

Chapter 3

The Cortical Monkey, Autoregulation and the Limbic-Spiritual State

Autoregulation is my term for a process by which an individual enters a natural healing energy state and then is guided by that energy to higher limbic-spiritual states. It is not about the popular—and, in my view, an entirely frivolous—notion of mind-over-body healing.

The terms *autoreg, autoregulation, self-regulation,* the *cortical* mode and the *limbic-spiritual state* appear throughout this volume. Below I briefly describe how these words took form and became part of my clinical vocabulary.

During my early years of practice of integrative medicine, I cared for many patients with severe chronic disorders. The use of prevailing drug therapies had failed to control their disorders and relieve their symptoms. I began clinical experiments with various approaches to stress control. Specifically, I focused on techniques that might be effective for slowing the heart rate, loosening up tightened arteries, warming cold hands and relaxing spastic muscles. In medical terminology, such body functions are considered part of the autonomic nervous system. It seemed logical to use the term autonomic regulation for such methods. My patients turned that into autoregulation, then abbreviated that to *autoreg.*

My early clinical experience also convinced me that my patients needed—and wanted—me to teach them effective methods for stress control and self-regulation as well as for facilitating natural healing. I recognized that many healing phenomena were clearly outside the domain of the autonomic nervous system, and my work extended far beyond any ideas of autonomic regulation. I also saw clearly the futility of the prevailing mind-over-body healing notions. It was evident to me that the prevailing notions of biofeedback with focus on one or more physiologic parameters were inadequate for my purpose.

It became obvious that healing is not an intellectual function. Rather, it is an energy phenomenon—and the energy of healing has almost nothing to do with the thinking mind. How do I convey this simple concept to my patients? I wondered. How do I introduce energy work in my very busy medical practice? Energy is a taboo in medicine, and energy healing is dismissed as voodoo medicine, unworthy of serious-minded men of medicine. How do I counter that? What language do I use to avoid being derided as a shaman or, worse, a charlatan. I searched for a simple term that would declare my purpose. During my meditation classes, I tried a number of terms for the healing energy state, but none very successfully except *limbic*. The limbic, of course, refers to the limbic system of the brain, which is generally associated with non-intellectual human experiences. To distinguish the healing limbic state from the disease-causing stressful state, I settled for the term cortical (see page 81 for explanation). Then I focused on the use of electrophysiologic equipment to observe how energy work demonstrably changes the energy patterns in their various body organs. The addition of moving, true-to-life computer graphs with sensor electrodes made it possible for me to effectively explain to my patients how their body organs worked, how diseases affect them, and how autoregulation can normalize distorted energy patterns.

THE MYSTERY AND MIRACLE OF HEALING

Further clinical work led me to conclude that the mystery—and the miracle—of healing was far too profound to be known by the superficial use of electrophysiologic equipment—nor can biologic profiles of various body organs prepared with such technology, no matter how true to life they might be, be of great value to someone serious about energy healing work. I realized that energy healing cannot be known at *any* plane by any of the prevailing notions of clever thinking—what psychologists and psychiatrists might regard as superior wisdom about unexpressed human emotions and hidden motives. I recognized that my own understanding of the healing phenomena, even after over three decades of intensive microscopic studies of injured and healing tissues, was pathetically inadequate.

In ending *The Cortical Monkey and Healing* published in 1990, I had written the following:

It seems improbable that man will ever fully understand the healing energy of love or, to be more precise, the healing energy of God. Medical technology, itself an expression of God's energy, is beginning to allow us to measure something about love, and then reproduce them. Measurement and reproducibility make up the language of science. One day, it seems, the men of medicine and the men of spirits will meet at some summit of union. The energy of God's love would have brought them together.

With passing years, own words written some years earlier took on altogether different meanings. The idea that a complete understanding of God's healing energy is clearly outside the reach of the human intellect struck me with uncommon energy. I recognized then that even an incomplete understanding of the mystery and the miracle of healing may not be achieved except in rare moments of resonance with the larger *presence* that permeates and surrounds each of us. That *presence* is not subordinate to our schedules. One has to patiently wait for those moments when the *organizing influence* of that *presence* reveals the mystery and the miracle of healing in ways that can only be *known* but never described.

My search for answers took a new turn: search for the meanings of healing turned into a search for ways of surrendering to that *organizing influence*. Then one day it occurred to me that that was the closest I would ever get to the knowledge of that healing energy: surrender and trust were going to be the operative words for me. A new term took form: the *limbic-spiritual*.

Looking back, my work with the very ill evolved through the following phases:

1. Stress management guided by the popular fight-or-flight concept of stress (which I now regard as frivolous and wholly irrelevant to my clinical work).
2. Focused autonomic regulation (which I now consider acceptable as long as it is seen as an intermediary state).
3. Unfocused self-regulation.
4. Meditation
5. Energy-over-mind healing energy.
6. Entry into the limbic-spiritual state.

The term limbic-spiritual, of course, remains an empty expression until a person finally has the good fortune to reach it. How does one ever know if one is in a limbic-spiritual state? One doesn't. One does not know when one is in it for the simple reason that in such a state there is no search, no discrimination, no judgment and no knowledge. There are only energetic perceptions. It is only when one returns from a limbic-spiritual state with altered perceptions and an altogether new knowledge of one's own condition that one begins to *know* that such states exist and may be reached. Here I do not refer to only profound mystical experiences that may or may not be translated into common language. Rather, I allude to degrees of enlightenment, which most individuals can know as parents, family members, friends, bakers, bankers, bosses, physicians, attorneys or plumbers. I do not speak here of Tibetan spirituality, rather of Manhattan spirituality—not of mysticism of Himalayan peaks, but of the mysticism of our garbage-strewn Main Streets, U.S.A.

The readers who know something about the path of meditation and the language of silence, of course, will readily understand what I write about here. For those who have not yet walked down that path, my patients speaking in this volume offer some guidance.

The staff at the Institute and I continue to use the term autoregulation in our self-regulation workshops for the new patients. But we all know that our work goes far beyond any ideas of self-healing—evidently a trivial and clinically irrelevant premise. *We know our work is about spirituality.*

The Cortical Monkey

I reproduce here one of my childhood memories from the companion volume, *The Cortical Monkey and Healing.*

There is a particular species of monkey native to Karnal, my birthplace. During my childhood, these monkeys lived in our town by the hundreds. They were a nuisance for the grown-ups, but for us children they were a lot of fun. I remember my father telling me how these monkeys had a peculiar habit. They did not let their wounds heal. If one of them ever lacerated his skin, he would pick at his wound continuously. He would peel off whatever little scab did form. These wounds festered for long periods of time.

PUTTING SOMETHING BETWEEN THE MONKEY AND HIS WOUND

It has occurred to me that the first man to invent a bandage probably got his idea from watching a monkey (or some other animal) constantly pick at his wound. It might have occurred to him that the way to let the wound heal would be to put something between the monkey and his wound. When he got hurt himself, the lesson learned from the monkey might have taken a practical turn. A bunch of leaves, perhaps of some herbal plant, might have served this purpose. This, or something similar, is likely to have been the forerunner of our modern Band-Aid.

There is something relevant in the story of Karnal monkeys to our ideas of self-regulation and healing. Time and again, I see patients who understand how their *cortical* condition throws roadblocks in the way of *limbic* healing. In our autoregulation laboratory, I demonstrate to them how their biologic profiles are composed of a host of electromagnetic or molecular events, I show them how their whole biology is sustained in an even state when they go limbic, and how it is thrown into turbulence when they go cortical. I explain to them the impact on their internal organs of *talking for control* and *listening for healing.* At intellectual and analytical levels, they seem to understand these phenomena. Yet, left to their own devices, they slide back into the calculating and competitive cortical state. They are unable to keep their analytical mind ("the cortical monkey") out of the way of the healing *limbic state.* Indeed, patient and persistent work is required to break long-established cortical habits and put the cortical monkey to sleep.

A decision I made during those early years of my clinical energy work was never to preach what I didn't practice myself. That meant I always had to test for myself each of the methods of autoregulation I considered for my patients. This personal experience—as well as the experiences of many patients who learned those methods well, became good "autoreggers," and related to me their experience—made it clear that it is extremely difficult, if at all possible, to enter the healing limbic-spiritual state without first dissolving the clutter of the thinking mind. Unrelenting thinking, I surmised, makes it impossible for anyone to be led by the gentle guiding energy of the limbic-spiritual state.

Thus, a simple and clinically valid conceptual model for incorporating self-regulation evolved in my mind. In this model, human biology exists in two basic but overlapping states: 1) a thinking state created and sustained by a superficial part of the brain—neocortex in scientific jargon—in which a person stays head-fixated, forever planning, forever scheming; and 2) a nonthinking energetic state in which the body tissues escape the tyranny of the thinking mind and revert to a natural healing state. I began to use the word cortical for the former and limbic-spiritual for the latter.

THE CORTICAL STATE

Thus, in autoregulation terminology, I used the term *cortical state* for a condition in which an individual thinks incessantly—and analyzes and censors himself endlessly. He craves for control on his life—and on the lives of those around him. Life becomes one continuous struggle of counting, computing and competing. His chronic thinking feeds upon itself, and he becomes addicted to thinking. The cortical monkey forever recycles past pain, and when that does not suffice, it precycles feared, future pain.

With its unrelenting chatter, the thinking mind relentlessly overdrives the physical body. It creates a Fourth-of-July chemistry, setting off thousands upon thousands of oxidative sparks in the body tissues. Simmering coals of anger and hostility are fanned and turned into leaping oxidative flames. This is not cheap melodrama. It is figuratively and literally accurate. The accelerated oxidative injury "cooks" the plasma proteins and "bakes" the cell membranes, just as heat cooks eggs. Anyone with basic training in the use of high-resolution, phase-contrast and dark-field microscope can test the validity of my statement. All he needs to do is to study a drop of blood from a chronically ill and highly stressed patient—just as I do every working day. Such oxidative cooking and baking of proteins and cells is not limited to blood cells. It affects proteins of all tissue fluids and cells of all body organs. Such accelerated oxidative stress shatters antioxidant defenses and batters various body organ ecosystems. This is how, at a fundamental level, diseases begin and perpetuate themselves.

THE LIMBIC-SPIRITUAL STATE

I use the term *limbic-spiritual state for* an individual's native state of spontaneous healing energy. The limbic-spiritual state "cares" and "comforts," coddling and soothing injured cells and tissues. This state creates and sustains healing environments for tissues in turmoil. Healing miracles simply follow. Again, this is not an empty play on words. I observe—and clearly document for my patients—such changes with suitable electrophysiologic equipment every week in my autoregulation laboratory. When the human frame is in a steady state, continuity of health-promoting basic life functions is assured. It keeps a heart's rhythm regular; arterial pulses even and full; breathing cycles slow and sustained; and other body organ functions in order.

In the healing context, the limbic-spiritual state allows a person to perceive the vibrant energy of living tissues and simply allows him to be guided by the transcendental wisdom of that energy. No effort is necessary in this state to make things happen—not even the healing phenomena. Of course, there is no room for any frivolous mind-over-body healing notions there. (Injured tissues—I'm certain—have no respect for our clever-thinking schemes for imposing healing on them.) These are not mere plays on words. Rather, these are simple conclusions drawn from personal experiences.

JOURNEY TO THE LIMBIC-SPIRITUAL

It is one thing for a physician to gain insights into some aspects of the healing phenomena he observes in his patients. It is an altogether different matter to incorporate into his clinical practice sound applications of those observations. Autoregulation is about perception of energy, and the limbic-spiritual state is an energy state. I saw the problem clearly. Unless my patients could experience some energy phenomena, I could not see significant clinical benefits. Furthermore, some individuals would be expected to experience the energy phenomena rather quickly, while others may require persistent efforts. Even under ideal conditions—and I gathered that from long hours of my own practice of autoregulation—such training must be accepted as a journey. And for the very sick who might need the limbic-spiritual most, this journey would be arduous and torturous. This would be serious business, and mere inspirational words won't work.

Another difficulty I repeatedly faced was the obvious paradox inherent in this work. Genuine autoregulation is a methodless activity. Yet, before most people can reach that state, they need training. So, I had to teach my patients several methods of autoregulation, and at the same time tell them that they would unlearn all that once they became good enough to do autoregulation methodlessly. How do I go about that? I wondered. Prepare them to learn and unlearn, and both at the same time?

Over the years these problems did resolve themselves. Not only did I begin to see things clearly myself, I found ways to explain these to my patients. Below, I include brief comments about some of my core concepts in this work.

HEALING IN THE LIMBIC-SPIRITUAL STATE IS NOT HEALING WITH COUNSELING, ANALYSIS, REGRESSION, HYPNOSIS OR BIOFEEDBACK

Compassion comforts. Love heals. The energy of prayer works. All that is self-evident. And it matters little whether compassion, love or prayers comes through a parent, a sibling, a friend, the clergy or some professional.

All methods that a professional uses to console a suffering individual are acceptable as long as the goal of short-term relief does not thwart the long-term recovery process. In my view, the very essence of limbic-spiritual healing is *knowing* the true nature of one's suffering. Such knowledge begins with the language of silence, and healing begins first at an intuitive-visceral plane, then at higher limbic-spiritual planes.

The journey to the limbic-spiritual takes a path that leads to freedom, and not dependence on someone else. As for those who provide guidance, the essence of that guidance is showing the way to independence. Thus, for the professional, the goal of all disease-reversal and recovery programs is to teach the patient ways of self-reliance—in matters of nutrition, environment, fitness, language of silence and energy perceptions. I consider it a failure on my part if I do not succeed in helping a patient see this clearly. I am a realist who has learned that long-suffering patients need enormous support before reaching the physical relief and clarity of vision for the insight I write about here.

Regrettably, counseling, analysis, regression, hypnosis and biofeedback—as they are often practiced today—sink the patient deeper and deeper into dependence on the therapist. In many cases, these therapies offer little more than cortical traps. Many of my patients received such therapies for years before they consulted me. It takes very little time and training for them to see the difference between talking for control and being guided by their energy for healing. Talking in most instances is a mere recycling of misery; the language of silence is liberating.

LIMBIC-SPIRITUAL HEALING, HYPNOTISM AND THE PLACEBO

There is one fundamental difference between the results obtained with a hypnotism and limbic-spiritual work: In a hypnotic trance, a person surrenders to the whims of the hypnotist while the limbic-spiritual path leads to surrender to the unknown. In hypnosis, a subject depends on the therapist and his dependance deepens with continued work; in the limbic-spiritual learns to trust—and be led by—the infinite mystery of the unknowable.

The placebo is a cruel deception. An ill-informed and arrogant professional seeks to establish control over his unsuspecting victim with a sugar pill which he passes as an effective remedy. A physician who prescribes a placebo is ill-informed because he really does not understand the essential healing power of the trust which a patient bestows upon his physician. What the patient expects from his physician is his (physician's) knowledge and experience dispensed as a medicine. What he gets is sheer deception. The physician with a placebo prescription is arrogant because he assumes he knows all there is to know—and that he is certain that there is nothing wrong with the patient. What amazes me is many of my colleagues continue to prescribe placebos.

Of course, sometimes the patient finds out that his physician is a trickster. He learns that what he thought was an effective remedy turns out to be a deliberate fraud on the part of the person he was willing to trust his health and life with. The patient under such circumstances is usually too disgusted with his physician to protest in words. There are some exceptions. I recall reading someplace about a man who shot and killed his oncologist when he found out his mother's cancer was treated with a placebo pill.

Neither the stupor created by the hypnotist nor the false promise created by an internist's sugar pill bring forth any insights into the true nature of a patient's suffering. In each case, the patient remains in the dark. Indeed, notwithstanding limited temporary benefits, both approaches further add to patient's distress at his ignorance of what ails him.

The promise of limbic-spiritual healing is different. It is profound insight and true enlightenment that comes through one's linkage with the larger *presence* that permeates and surrounds him at all times. There is no intermediary in this linkage. There is no possibility of deception or illusion there. It is true that limbic-spiritual healing cannot be procured on short order, but its great boon is that its benefits endure.

I illustrate this essential difference by citing an example: A physician gives his patient a placebo (sugar capsule) and tells him that the medicine in the capsule will cure his headache. The placebo works, and the headache indeed is relieved. Because the patient in this case was tricked into thinking that the sugar capsule in the placebo was an effective remedy, it added nothing to his understanding of the true nature of his affliction. On those occasions when the patient discovers the truth, he is deeply disappointed and naturally feels victimized by his physician.

A hypnotist hypnotizes a patient suffering from a migraine headache to relieve his pain. The hypnotic suggestion works, and the headache is relieved. The patient associates the hypnotic trance with some sort of a spell, albeit a helpful and healthful spell. This patient is not much better than the one enjoying the placebo effect, insofar as his understanding of the true nature of things is obscured. In both cases, the patient learns to depend on the therapist. With each migraine, the dependence grows while the benefits of the therapy diminish. I have seen no exceptions.

I do not write this to deny possible temporary benefits of hypnosis, nor to discourage anyone from its use. At times even minimal symptom relief can be a blessing, and hypnosis can provide relief without any toxicity. But I do not accept it as a legitimate long-term approach to chronic suffering. Self-regulation, and self-regulation alone, can take us to the gates of the spiritual world which we must enter on our own. It is that spiritual world that gives us enduring relief from the suffering caused by disease.

**LIMBIC-SPIRITUAL HEALING
IS AN ENERGY-OVER-MIND PHENOMENA**

Autoregulation, I wrote earlier in this chapter, is a process by which an individual enters a limbic-spiritual state and is guided by its gentle energy. Once in that state, one simply surrenders to that energy, allowing oneself to be guided by that gentle healing energy.

All living beings—cells, tissues and body organs—are energy beings. Here I do not speak in a metaphysical sense. Rather, I state a self-evident fact. In autoregulation, we simply allow ourselves to be guided by the innate energy of living beings. Before we can do that, however, we need to learn how to perceive the patterns of energy in our tissues, whether healthy or sick.

In my clinical work, I use electromagnetic technology to evaluate true-to-life energy patterns in the various body organs. With suitable computer technology, it is now possible to demonstrate to my patients both the disease-causing cortical and healing limbic-spiritual energy patterns. Such technology is very valuable in understanding how the way we look at the world around us changes our entire biologic profiles—how our energy patterns change when we successfully banish the thinking mind and allow ourselves to be led by such energy. Machines do not heal—and biofeedback technology is no exception. There is, however, considerable value in demonstrating objective, measurable, and reproducible electromagnetic changes during autoregulation. The technology clearly documents that the energy patterns in the health—disease continuum are real. It appeases the cortical monkey by giving it a taste of its own medicine.

SCIENCE CATCHES UP WITH EMPIRICISM

I consider a physician's life an enormous privilege. Indeed, such is my profound gratitude at being allowed to do my clinical work—or perhaps it is simply a matter of a severely limited view of life—that I am never comfortable contemplating another line of work if I were to live a second life. I sometimes wonder if I were to have a chance to live at any time in history, what time would that be? It would be now.

This is a wondrous time for those who treasure both the healing philosophy of the ancients and the promise of 21st-century medical technology. The ancients understood well the essential nature of the healing process: its spontaneity, range and completeness when it is permitted to follow its natural course. Unable to explore the inner workings of the human body, they focused on providing ingredients and environment for healing. Along the way they gained enormous insights into the mystery and miracle of the healing phenomena. Our Star Wars technology now allows us to test the scientific basis of their intuitive insights. It is a matter of unending amazement for me to see how science catches up with empiricism.

In *Rats* I wrote about my vision for the medicine of the future: Given informed choice, people will prefer therapies based on the physics of health rather than on the chemistry of disease.

Certainly I find that true of my own clinical work.

Specifically, I can now observe the inner workings of the human body—at the levels of individual body organs, tissues, cells, even molecules—in ways that was unimaginable when I entered medical school four decades ago. For example, in my practice I take a drop of blood from my patients and use a high-resolution microscope to observe evidence of oxidative damage to living blood cells and plasma proteins. I can directly see how effective or ineffective immune cells are in their defense functions. I can directly look at yeast and other microbes in the blood stream and recognize the extent of devastation caused by them—I can see how dirty or clean the blood of my patient is. I published some photomicrographs showing such damage in the companion volume *RDA: Rats, Drugs and Assumptions.* (Blood cells and plasma proteins do not lie. Cells and enzymes of chronic fatigue sufferers—human canaries as I call them—always tell the truth. Uninformed doctors who consider chronic fatigue an all-in-the-head problem should sometimes look at the blood cells of their patients.)

I use an electrodermal conductance technology to observe directly how various foods can affect my patient's energy patterns, then use that knowledge to guide my patients for optimal food choices to reverse chronic food-related disorders and restore health. I provided much useful information about this subject in *The Butterfly and Life Span Nutrition.*

In my autoregulation laboratory I use computerized electrophysiologic equipment to study how regular or irregular rhythms of the various body organs are for a given patient. An early lesson I learned from my patients was that the only part of the human condition that lies is the mind. The heart, arteries, muscle and skin tissues never learned how to lie. So it seemed natural to me that I should ignore the thinking mind in matters of healing energy work. I addressed this subject and published pictures of some electrophysiologic profiles in limbic and cortical modes in *The Cortical Monkey and Healing.*

Below, I reproduce some text from the companion volume *RDA: Rats, Drugs and Assumptions* to elaborate some core concepts in my work.

POSITIVE THINKING, NO MATTER HOW CLEVER, IS OF LIMITED VALUE IN HEALING

Another lesson I learned from my patients in those early years was that the common advice of positive thinking is a cruel joke on the severely ill. As desirable as positive thinking may seem on the surface, it is still thinking—and thinking, no matter how clever, cannot heal. My work with very ill patients convinced me that positive thinking is not sufficient to transform one's perturbed biology from a cortical, disease-causing state to a calm, healing, energetic, limbic-spiritual state. I recognized that it was cruel to advise patients to think positively when they were in the throes of intense suffering.

On the following pages, I illustrate some electromagnetic patterns of tissue energy which I commonly observe in my patients during autoregulation training. In the biologic profiles shown below, I illustrate stressful and disease-causing cortical profiles as well as some changes in such patterns when an individual escapes the tyranny of the mind and is guided to the limbic-spiritual state.

The biologic profile given below illustrates a disease-causing cortical mode of the functions of various body organs. The sensing electrodes attached to the patient indicate electromagnetic expressions of spasm of the arteries (single arrow), stress on the heart as shown by wide swings in the heart rate (two arrows), and a high skin conductance (three arrows).

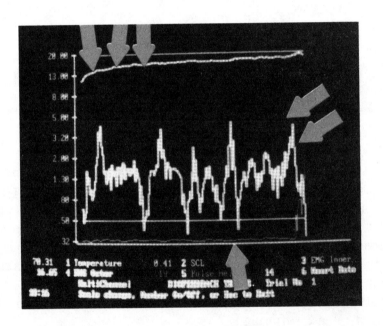

The biologic profile given below illustrates a healing limbic mode of function of various body organs. The sensor electrodes indicate electromagnetic expressions of natural, unstrained functions of arteries (bottom line), muscles (top two line), the heart (bright line, third from top), and skin conductance energy (faint line that can be seen in some places below the nearly straight bottom line).

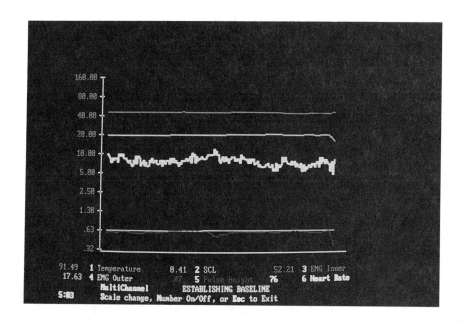

The biologic profile given below illustrates how a restful, healing limbic mode during autoregulation turns into a stressful, disease-causing cortical mode when autoregulation is interrupted. Note how the graph lines representing functions of arteries, muscles, the heart and skin abruptly change in the left side of the profile. The arteries go into a spasm almost immediately when autoregulation ends, the heart responds to tightened arteries after a brief delay, and skin conductance rises. With continued practice of autoregulation, the healing limbic mode persists even when the person is asked to perform any function—one learns to *live* in the limbic mode.

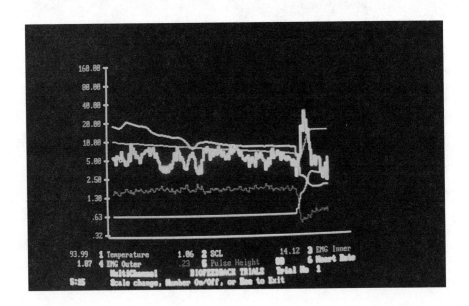

IT'S TOO SIMPLE

Ken Gerdes, M.D., of Denver, an internist and a close friend, was among the group of physicians who attended my first autoregulation workshop for physicians in 1987. He wrote to me on his way back to Denver. He thought my discussion on the molecular basis of aging, accelerated aging, potential for intervention and treatment of disease with autoregulation was rational, logical and scientifically sound. Further, he had no difficulty accepting the clinical results that I was seeing with my autoregulation methods. "I have been thinking about it all day," he wrote. "I am troubled about one thing. It's too simple."

During the first two years of my work with autoregulation, I was also troubled, sometimes deeply troubled, about the utter simplicity of the principles and practice of autoregulation. As I closely observed more and more of my patients resolve their various chronic diseases without drugs, I recognized I had to make a choice:

I could dismiss as apocryphal the accounts of my patients (consider them naive, or worse, deceitful) and stop my work in self-regulation.

Or,

I could accept self-regulation as a valid medical discipline that gives us predictable clinical results and continue my work to advance this field.

I chose the second option.

After I gave my very first autoregulation workshop for physicians, three of the 14 physicians from this group incorporated autoregulation in their clinical practice. After each subsequent workshop, I received calls from physicians affirming the benefits of one or more features of autoregulation.

This ongoing peer review is most valuable to me. It sustains me during many periods of self-doubt and discouragement.

THE WAY WE LOOK AT THE WORLD AROUND
US DETERMINES WHAT OUR ENERGETIC
PATTERNS UNDER THE SKIN ARE

Every week my staff and I spend about three hours with a group of my patients in my autoregulation laboratory. I recommend that all my new patients consider three training sessions with me. In the laboratory, I wire them to various electronic sensors to monitor the energetic patterns of their skin, muscles, arteries and heart. That allows me to study the patterns of electromagnetic energy in their various body organs. It also allows me to help them understand how their body organs cope with stress, and how their energy patterns are normalized when they learn to escape the relentless censor of the thinking mind. At an intellectual level it is all so easy to understand. But healing, as I wrote earlier, is not an intellectual function. We need to enter higher states of energy and consciousness to truly break the chains of the thinking mind.

The way we look at the world around us determines the state of energy we are in. It is when we evade the ceaseless demands of the thinking mind that the body tissues return to their native state of healing energy.

NAMING WITHOUT KNOWING, KNOWING WITHOUT NAMING

The thinking mind thrives on naming things—names are crutches of the cortical monkey. Without names it is disoriented, unable to cope, exposed, and vulnerable. In my autoregulation training, I use some time-honored methods of naming things and then letting the names go. In the beginning, my patients often find this very confusing. Unable to latch on to any names, the cortical monkey becomes disoriented, then settles down as the names of things lose their grip. The energy states change and there are limbic periods when perceptions of tissue energy sublimate cortical thoughts. With training, such periods grow longer until a person reaches a state when she recognizes the state she was in only when she comes out of it. Then she *knows* the order of things in human energy dynamics: the relationship of the mind with the body (the mind punishes tissues by its ceaseless chatter) and the relationship of tissue energy with the mind (the energy of living tissues shuts up the thinking mind).

We begin by naming things we do not know and end up knowing things we cannot name.

WHEN THE DIAGNOSIS BECOMES A KILLER

Many of my patients arrive with thick bundles of medical records, having seen multiple physicians before me. As I thumb through their records, I see the many different diagnoses made by previous physicians. Such patients carry a big burden of uncertainty as to the nature of their illness. Each time they are told that a diagnosis has been firmly established they are expected to respond to the *drug of choice*. And each time, the miracle drug fails them. The dogma of drug medicine holds that precise diagnoses are essential for drug regimens to work. This is, of course, where the real problem starts.

In chronic illness the name of the disease is not important. Recognition and management of the biological burdens that increase oxidant stress on tissues and damage antioxidant and immune defenses are the relevant issues. So my primary task is to help the patient understand the nature of oxidant stresses and the dynamics of the healing phenomenon. I need to help them break free from the disease model of thinking that holds back the healing response. The task of addressing all relevant issues of nutrition, environment, stress and fitness becomes much easier for the patient once those chains are broken.

Autoregulation—energy healing with a sound knowledge of biologic-oxidative stressors—is extremely valuable, both for the patient and his physician. This approach allows both to see the energetic-molecular basis of illness clearly. This is an honest approach without any need for the physician to hide behind meaningless diagnostic labels. For the patient, it underscores the futility of shopping for diagnosis when his resources are scarce.

GIVING THE CORTICAL MONKEY A DOSE OF HIS OWN MEDICINE

Patients often ask me why autoreg is not mind-over-body healing. Don't we use the mind to do autoregulation?

When we *begin* autoregulation, indeed, we use the thinking mind. So the simple sentences that someone in autoregulation training learns may be regarded as a mental activity. However, the purpose of those sentences is not to use the mind to heal the body. Rather, it is to reach a state in which the thinking mind is stilled, and perceptions of tissue energy lead us into deeper energy states that effectively exclude mental chatter.

When I do autoregulation—and I do so frequently during my work in the laboratory and clinic—I do not use the steps I teach my patients in autoregulation classes. I do not follow any technique. After years of training and teaching autoregulation, I have reached a state where perceptions of energy come to me spontaneously, without uttering any sentences or employing any of the other methods I teach others. Almost instantaneously, I perceive the energy in my tissue, then there is nothing more for me to do.

The gentle guiding energy does the rest. On rare occasions, when I am extremely rushed or a captive of my thinking mind, the energy perceptions do not arrive readily. At such times, I—like my patients—rely on limbic breathing or simple sentences to quell my screaming mind so that the healing energy can prevail. Many of my patients relate similar personal experiences after long hours of such work. Indeed, all good autoregulators reach that stage when words or techniques are irrelevant to autoregulation.

The essential point here is that autoregulation is not about mind-over-body healing. It is the exact opposite: an energy-over-mind state that brings profound visceral-energetic stillness—a stillness that is too deep for words. That is the limbic-spiritual state.

DO MIND-OVER-BODY APPROACHES
REALLY WORK?

Notwithstanding the rather limited and temporary benefits of positive thinking and affirmation, I have seen no evidence that mind-over-body approaches to healing work. In contrast, energy-over-mind approaches heal. I observe evidence of that every Wednesday evening during self-regulation training sessions. When the clutter of the thinking mind is put to rest, the energy that constitutes us is free to guide us.

Our infatuation with mind-over-body healing is a relatively recent development. Since man became aware of the healing response in injured tissues, he has been interested in the energy phenomenon. Since antiquity, people have explored the various dimensions of the healing phenomenon, and have entertained the question of how to facilitate a natural healing response in injured tissues. To date, I can find no records showing that the ancients ever succeeded in using their minds to order healing in tissues. I have never seen convincing evidence from any faith healers, mystics, shamans, or modern gurus of the mind-over-body industry indicating that they found a way *to use their thinking minds to prod the nonhealing tissues to heal*—at least in the physical ways that can be *observed* with a microscope or assessed by other chemical and physical means.

This is not to say that miracles do not happen. I *know* they happen. I have seen miracles take place among my patients thousands of times. But miracles are energy phenomena. I have yet to see proof that miracles can be brought about by clever thinking.

CAN THE MIND COAX INJURED TISSUES TO HEAL QUICKER, OR DO TISSUES HEAL FASTER WHEN THE MIND IS STILLED?

In many well-documented cases, the course of illness appears to have been radically altered by certain measures taken by the sick. The question that intrigues me is whether the observed benefits resulted because the mind ordained the injured tissues to heal or because injured tissues were spared the disease-promoting activities of the thinking mind. Do diseased tissues regenerate more expediently when they are relentlessly driven by schemes concocted by the thinking mind? Or do they heal more quickly when the unrelenting mind is stilled? Before the thinking mind can heal hurt tissues, it must first understand how healing occurs. For the mind to fix a healing problem, it must first know what that healing problem is. The issue is not that the phenomenon of healing can be facilitated. It clearly can be. The question is what, if any, role does the thinking mind play in the healing response? It amuses me that those who speak the loudest of their mind's ability to heal are the people who seem to have the least understanding of the observable healing response in distressed tissues.

"IT JUST HAPPENS, DR. ALI, HONEST, IT JUST HAPPENS"

A very large number of patients tell me they can control migraine attacks, asthma episodes, colitis and other disorders with mind-over-body healing. Some tell me that they can heal chronically painful backs with their minds. Such stories are of intense interest to me. I never doubt that these people are telling me the truth. What I pursue vigorously is *how* they use their minds to heal the body. How do they persuade their tightened arteries to let go so that they might get some relief from migraine pain? How do they plead with, coax or simply order their spastic bronchial tubes to open so they can breathe without using drugs? How do they convince their ulcerated colons to cease from episodes of cramping and bleeding? How do they use their minds to tell irritated, rebellious muscles in their backs to loosen up?

To date no one has ever answered such questions. When questioned, my patients become defensive, making statements such as:

"Dr. Ali, I can often control my asthma attacks," the patient proudly tells me.
"That's wonderful! How do you do it?" I ask.
"You know how, don't you?"
"No, I really don't."
"Well, with mind control." He smiles.
"Tell me how you do mind control."
"With mind-over-body healing."

"How do you do your mind-over-body healing?" I persist.

"You know! The mind-over-body approach." He becomes a little tentative.

"Tell me how you do your mind-over-body approach to asthma?" I press him. "I mean, how do you use your mind to send messages to the bronchial tubes to open so that air can get in?"

"Well..." The patient stops in midsentence.

"Yes..." I coax him.

"I... I... I don't know how..."

"Just think about it. Try to recall how you do your mind-over-body thing. I'm very interested in that."

"It just happens, Doc."

"Of course, it happens. But I need to understand how it happens. If you can teach me how you do it, then I can teach your method to my other patients who suffer from asthma."

"It just happens, Dr. Ali, honest, it just happens."

"Of course, it does!" I reassure him.

"You really don't believe me, do you?" he asks.

"Of course I do," I assert. "Every Wednesday I spend three hours with my patients teaching them self-regulation. So I do know it works. I just want to know how *you* do it."

"Maybe I can't explain it, but it *does* work."

"I know! I know! I don't doubt you for one moment."

"So you do believe mind-over-body works?"

"I didn't say that, did I? It would have been different if we really could use our minds to do such things. But how do we know it is the working of the mind if the mind does not even know what it is? How can we say we use our mind to do something our mind doesn't even understand?"

"How else do you think it works?"

"I don't know. Perhaps because you have intuitively found a way to shut off your thinking mind—keep the cortical monkey out. Perhaps because tissue energy shuts out the mind so that the natural healing state of energy in injured tissues can do what Nature designed it to do—heal. Perhaps because the natural state of the bronchial tubes is to stay relaxed and open. That's what they do when they are left alone—when the ceaseless demands of their thinking minds are blocked by the healing energy of irritated bronchial tubes. Isn't that what asthma sufferers tell us? Stress makes their asthma worse."

"You mean it is not the mind that heals? It's something else? Something other than my thinking mind?" he asks, perplexed.

"Isn't that what you just told me?" I retort.

THE MIND OF AN OSTEOBLAST

Fractured bones heal without taking cues from the thinking mind. To my knowledge, osteoblasts—the bone cells that multiply and lay down new bone for the healing of fractured bones—do not have much respect for mind-over-body healing.

Consider wounds healing in healthy little children, vigorous adults and active elderly individuals. Suppose a two-year-old girl, a 42-year-old woman and a 92-year-old woman trip over a stone and fracture their wrist bones. Whose broken bones will heal the fastest and whose will take the longest? Predictably, the child's broken bones will heal in the shortest time and the elderly woman's will take the longest. Now let us factor in the conventional mind-over-body approach. The child does not even know that such notions as mind-over-body healing exist, makes no attempt to engage in it, and yet her bones heal the quickest. The 92-year-old woman should have the most knowledge and should have all the necessary time to put to use her mind-over-body healing skills. Yet, she will have the most difficulty and, in most instances, can be expected to have incomplete bone healing even under ideal circumstances. How do we reconcile these everyday observations with the mind-over-body theory?

The osteoblast cells in the two-year-old girl burst into activity and merrily go about their business of mending broken bones, following their own energy signals, totally oblivious of what her mind may or may not dictate. Cells revved up with healing energy cherish their autonomy. The healing cells in the 42-year-old woman will follow a different pace and heal the bone slowly. The osteoblast cells of the 92-year-old woman will lay out new bone in their own leisurely way, sensing no need to acknowledge any of the exhortations of the clever, thinking mind.

NONUNION IN PEOPLE, MALUNION IN ANIMALS

As a young surgeon in training, first in Pakistan and later in England, I saw many cases of nonunion of fractured bones. Nonunion refers to a condition in which fractured bones do not heal even when set and immobilized in a cast. For some reasons, the natural healing process is arrested in this condition. (Impaired blood circulation, poor nutritional status and prolonged immobilization are some of the causes of nonunion.) Malunion refers to cases in which the two broken ends of the bone unite, but do so in a crooked way.

The subject of nonunion often summons references to the healing phenomena in primitive cultures and in wild animals.

Fractured bones heal among tribal cultures in which broken bones are set and splinted without using modern technology, though the broken bones often heal with malunion—in a malaligned fashion. Similarly, fractured bones always heal in the animal kingdom, though predictably producing crookedly healed bones. Nonunion is a rare phenomenon in nature. By contrast, nonunion is not very uncommon after the broken bones are immobilized in casts. Thus, there is a clear distinction between healing of fractured bone under natural circumstances with minimal or no interference and healing of broken bones under conditions of forced immobilization with orthopedic techniques. Nonunion is a price we pay for introducing the mind of man to the natural healing response in bone.

Obviously, I do not make a case here for not using modern orthopedic techniques on fractured bones. I do not advocate that we accept crookedly healed bones. I include here brief comments about the conditions of nonunion and malunion of fractured bones to illustrate my essential point: The thinking mind cannot force healing on osteoblast cells. These cells will do what Nature designed them to do. They lay down new bone and mold and remold such bone in response to healthy stresses of life so that the end result is a healed bone. Children's broken bones usually heal quickly. The mended bones model and remodel themselves continuously. X-rays of such bones, taken several months after the healing response began, show perfect bone structure so that someone unfamiliar with the case would not even suspect that a fracture had occurred. The thinking mind clearly plays no role in such bone healing.

My essential point in this brief discussion of bone healing is that while the mind can interfere with bone healing, it cannot initiate or speed the healing response in broken bones.

THE ADRENALINE PUMP
AND THE MIND OF A GAZELLE

Nature gave us the fight-or-flight response as a survival technique. When the mind perceives a threat, a large number of reflex reactions—outside the mind's control—gear the body for response. The heart races to pump more blood for maximal effort; the lungs hyperventilate to inhale more oxygen to sustain the effort; the pupils dilate to see more; and the muscles are held taut for maximum efficiency. The fight-or-flight response is elicited by bursts of adrenaline from the adrenal gland.

A leopard crouches behind the bush and slowly approaches a gazelle grazing in a meadow. When the leopard can no longer hide its approach, it lunges forward toward the gazelle. The prey sees a flashing image, freezes for a moment in shock, then breaks into a frenzied dash. The flashing image has been processed by the gazelle. Almost instantly an adrenaline surge sends a barrage of molecular messages that thrust the body into a dance of survival. Some minutes later, the exhausted leopard gives up the chase, and the gazelle escapes. Within moments, the chemistry of the gazelle begins its return to a normal state, as the adrenaline peak ebbs and the related flight molecules break down. Does the gazelle use its mind to control its body and return its Fourth-of-July chemistry to a health-restoring steady state of energy?

THE MIND CREATES, BUT HEALING ENERGY PUTS OUT THE OXIDATIVE FLAMES OF THE FOURTH-OF-JULY CHEMISTRY

The mind can light up the oxidative sparks of anger, resentment and hostility, but the clever designs of the thinking mind cannot extinguish such sparks. I see evidence of this phenomenon every working day. An occupied mind—the cortical monkey in autoregulation lingo—loves to recycle misery. It thrives on packaging and repackaging past hurts. When that is not enough, it precycles feared, future misery. It turns a natural state of healing energy into turbulent Fourth-of-July chemistry. It mercilessly drives the energy enzyme pathways of the body, literally short-circuiting human energy systems. Unable to cope with the unending demands of the thinking mind, the energy-depleted and exhausted tissues succumb. The clever-thinking mind succeeds in its relentless pursuit. In *What Do Lions Know About Stress?* I address the subject at length and make many specific suggestions for putting out the oxidative flames that fan the Fourth-of-July chemistry.

EARLY MAN AND THE BODY-MIND-SPIRIT TRIO

I am fascinated by the ancient records of spiritual healing. In all cultures and in all segments of mankind's history, there is clear evidence of spiritual healing. Methods change, but the essence of healing does not. It is also clear that such healing was always an energy phenomenon, though its essential nature escaped critical intellectual scrutiny—as it continues to do to date. If spiritual healing is hocus-pocus—as my colleagues in drug medicine believe—how could it survive for millennia? Fads in medicine come and go. Why did the essential mystery of spiritual healing endure?

How did early man come up with his body-mind-spirit trio in the first place? It is easy to understand why he thought about the first two. He had bodily senses, and he could think, imagine, hope and dream. But why the third element? How did he know that the third element of the spirit existed? After all, whatever he could think about or imagine comes under the jurisdiction of the mind. No matter how wide the swing of his imagination or how vast the reach of his mind, it was all an intellectual function. How did he dream up the very notion that the spirit existed? Indeed, the very thought of the spirit is well within the confines of the thought process. By definition, the spirit must be accepted as beyond our physical senses and beyond all intellectual faculties.

The primitive healer closed his eyes and went into an altered energy state for the healing ritual. The shaman of today does the same. Closed eyes and the rhythm of the drums allowed the ancient to escape the confines of the thinking mind. It is the same with the shaman and others who take this healing approach.

MUSIC AND HEALING

Music sustains. Music alleviates suffering. Music heals. How does music do all that? How does music reverse a disease process?

Is musical transformation an intellectual function? Did Mozart and Beethoven engage in highly intellectual functions when they composed? I doubt if any singer in the history of mankind has been listened to more frequently than the Indian singer, Lata Mangeshkar. It has been estimated that more than a billion and a half people in India, Pakistan, Bangladesh, Far East, Middle East, South Africa and many other countries listen to her songs regularly. Certainly, Lata is heard more frequently in New York City taxis than any other singer. (More than 80 percent of the taxis in the city are driven by Pakistanis and Indians.) Lata has the singular quality of reaching the core of her listeners. I doubt if any singer has ever alleviated more human suffering with her/his words than Lata has. Does she use her mind to exert her healing influence? Or does she harness the mental faculties of her listeners to order their injured tissues to shape up—and heal themselves? "Man, if you gotta ask you'll never know," Louis Armstrong replied when asked what jazz is. Thomas (Fats) Waller spoke of the same dimension when asked to explain rhythm: "Lady, if you got to ask you ain't got it." Healing, like music and rhythm, cannot be explained or understood—it can only be *known*. The gurus of the mind-over-body industry do not seem to know this.

WHY ARE WE PHYSICIANS MIFFED BY THE MIND-OVER-BODY APPROACH TO HEALING?

This is an interesting question. Physicians make their living treating diseases, but their sincerity is widely questioned in the U.S. today. Notwithstanding such cynicism, a vast majority of physicians are hard-working, caring and compassionate professionals. Physicians *do* want their patients to get better. What could be safer, less expensive and convenient than mind-over-body healing for physicians? Unfortunately, most physicians are too wedded to drug medicine to reflect on this simple question.

Most advances of Star Wars medicine took place in the later part of this century. Before that, we physicians had none of the high-tech tools of our trade. It would have been the most natural thing for us to engage in the mind-over-body healing approach. So why didn't we?

It may be argued that physicians were not seduced by mind-over-body healing because it would have disempowered them—put the patient in charge of the healing process. It would have minimized the importance of the physician's role in the care of the sick, and it might have denigrated their herbs and lancets. Indeed, implicit was the clear risk that success in mind-over-body healing might put them out of commission. There is, however, a problem with this theory. Clearly, there were physicians in the past whose commitment to the well-being of their patients was unequivocally sufficient to consider this approach—if for no other reason than that mind-over-body healing has no serious adverse effects.

So why didn't physicians engage mind-over-body healing? I believe the real answer is that they found it simply doesn't work—notwithstanding rather limited benefits of positive thinking and affirmations of health. Even in modern times, we have known that what is being touted as mind-over-body techniques are petty intellectual games.

There is another interesting aspect to this subject. If mind-over-body healing really worked, we physicians would have known this better than any other group. We would have certainly adopted the method for personal use and for treating our family members. The reality is quite different: We physicians, as a group, probably use more drugs for our own infirmities than any other large group of professionals. If the mind-over-body approach really worked, certainly we, more than any other group, would have put it into personal use.

Injured molecules, cells and tissues heal spontaneously when they are spared the clever healing schemes of the thinking mind. I discuss this simple truth that perceptive individuals in the healing profession have known for thousands of years at length in the companion volume *The Cortical Monkey and Healing*.

PSYCHOSOMATIC AND SOMATOPSYCHIC MODELS OF DISEASE ARE ARTIFACTS OF OUR THINKING

Diseases are burdens on biology. Human intellect and human body organs are integral parts of the human condition. To separate them, as Socrates lamented, is to negate the completeness of the human condition.

Our technology has rendered irrelevant the debate on the psychosomatic and somatopsychic nature of diseases. Advances in behavioral biology and experimental psychology have put these two disciplines on a collision course; a complete merger between the two is simply a matter of time.

Hope is an energetic-molecular event. So is dejection. Neuropeptide research is closing in on defining emotions and behavior as chemical sequences. The French philosopher, Teilhard de Chardin, dreamed of the day when man's technology would conquer oceans and winds and begin to explore the energy of love. We are seeing the dawn of that day.

Energy healing in limbic-spiritual states—the energy-over-mind approach—brings forth profound and demonstrable changes in human biology. Clinically, many of my patients can control asthma and arthritis, lower blood pressure in hypertension, and normalize overactive and underactive thyroid glands with consistency and predictability. It is unusual for me to see a patient who is unable to learn how to alter one or more electrophysiologic responses during his very first training session with me in our autoregulation laboratory.

I have not seen the mind-over-body gospel work. The clinical benefits of the positive-thinking gospel which I have observed myself have been very limited—hardly worth the effort. The energy-over-mind approach—and the limbic-spiritual state it seeks to reach—often is difficult for patients with serious chronic illnesses. However, this approach does work, and many of my patients do reverse their diseases when they finally succeed in energy healing work. They enthusiastically tell me about the clinical benefits of canceling the cortical clutter. When the cortical monkey finally shuts up, injured tissues heal. Tissues evidently know their business.

I began this chapter by saying that healing is an energy function—and that it is a natural state of energy. I close this chapter now by returning to it. The essence of self-regulation is in achieving a healing energy state—when the energy of body tissue guides us. It is a state in which we banish the thinking mind. Autoregulation, guided by healing energy, ends the ceaseless chatter of the mind that relentlessly beats up on injured tissues. *It is a process by which one reaches that limbic-spiritual state in which one simply surrenders to the gentle guiding energy of the presence that permeates and surrounds each of us at all times.*

*None of are victims. All of us are victims.
There is a canary within each of us, only
the cages look different. Each of us can fly
out.*

*Regret is a thief—it steals life. A life of
regret is a life stolen before it arrives.*

The Canary and Chronic Fatigue

Chapter 4

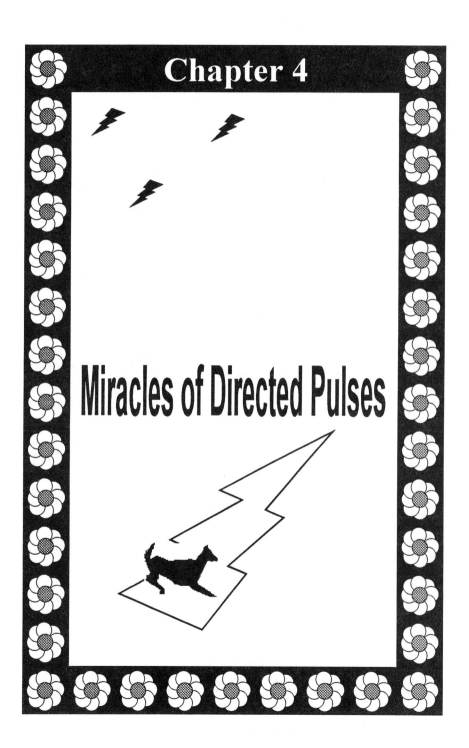

Miracles of Directed Pulses

*What is the hardest of all? That which you
hold the most simple; seeing with your own
eyes what is spread out before you.*

Goethe

The heart beats to pump blood into the arteries. Then it
relaxes and its chambers open up to receive blood from the veins.
During systole (the contraction phase of the heart), the pressure of
the blood in the arteries rises suddenly, creating a peak pressure.
During diastole (the relaxation phase of the heart), the pressure of
the blood within the arteries falls, creating a trough. The
difference between the high (systolic) and low (diastolic) pressures
creates a wave effect in the arteries that can be palpated at the
wrist, feet, neck and other areas in the body.

Under ordinary conditions, we are not aware of pulses in
our arteries. I coined the term *directed pulses* (the "pulses") to
describe a method by which a person can sense pulses in the
arteries in any given part of his body. I use this as the first step in
my autoregulation training for all patients.

What do pulses feel like? Most people have experienced the
throbbing sensation with headaches, tooth abscesses or inflamed
tissues. Of course, in such circumstances the throbbing sensation is
associated with pain of varying degrees. The pulses are also felt as
a throbbing sensation that follows the rhythm of the heart but is not

uncomfortable. Indeed, the experience of the pulses is very calming for the novice and deeply comforting for the experienced.

HEALING ENERGY

Autoregulation, as I define it earlier in this volume, is a process by which a person enters the natural state of healing energy. Once the energy of the pulses—or tissue energy in other forms—is perceived, one simply allows oneself to be guided by that energy. Perception of tissue energy might seem improbable to those who have never practiced self-regulation. In fact, it can be experienced physically, not merely understood intellectually, and it is easy to learn and simple to understand once one learns effective methods of self-regulation. Indeed, it is rare for me to see a patient who does not succeed in sensing the essential energy of his living tissues in the very first training session.

For more than 10 years, I have taught self-regulation to all my patients regardless of the nature of their illnesses. In these sessions, I introduce the principles and practices of self-regulation in basic terms. In my autoregulation laboratory, I use electrodes to monitor the energy levels and functions of the various body organs. The data are then fed into a computer that formats the information into easily understandable, multicolored, moving graphs on the computer screen.

Extensive clinical experience has convinced me that this training is the most valuable method for teaching patients to become aware of the energy patterns of living tissues. I advise my patients to follow up on the training with autoregulation, using tapes that I prepared specifically for this purpose. (The text of the basic autoregulation tape appears at the end of this chapter.) After initial training, the use of the tapes becomes unnecessary.

VISCERAL RESISTANCE

Earlier in my autoregulation work, I observed that some patients slide effortlessly into deep meditative states. These patients showed clear electrophysiological evidence of profound and demonstrable changes in the function of various body organs. Others found autoregulation hard to understand and its practice difficult. It appears the patients in the second group had some "visceral" resistance, an internal impediment to the practice of autoregulation that they could neither explain nor overcome.

Whereas the first group succeeded in regulating some of their biologic functions with just one or two training sessions, those in the second group required extensive training with several sessions to learn even the basic steps. After several unsuccessful attempts, some of them gave up autoregulation. The reason why some succeeded so readily while others failed, even after considerable effort, puzzled me. I searched for some simple method of teaching patients how to dissolve their internal, visceral resistance in order to perceive their tissue energy, an essential step if autoregulation is to succeed.

Intellectually, sensing tissue energy with autoregulation is a simple concept. However, it is unsettling for most physicians who have no real sense of the energy of living tissues. Often they contemptuously dismiss all references to energy in healing as witchcraft and sorcery. This is regrettable. All matter is condensed energy. This is elementary physics, not an abstract metaphysical notion. Living tissues are energy beings. (Indeed, from such a perspective of energy dynamics, nonliving entities such as stones are also energy entities: There is no difference between a grain of sand and a sandfly—both are energy beings.) Thus, whether a person can or cannot sense energy in his tissues is a matter of knowledge and training, and not that of witchcraft or sorcery.

HAND WARMING

Hand warming is one of the oldest, simplest, and most widely practiced methods of self-regulation. It is especially suitable for beginners. The warming of hands is easily sensed by the subject. The changed skin temperature of hands can be monitored and documented readily with inexpensive thermometers or suitable electronic devices. Beginners often have initial self-doubts. But the objective evidence of significant temperature changes effectively dispels any doubt about whether the beginner is really witnessing a true change or simply imagining it.

The hand-warming method generally worked well for most of my patients during the early years of my work with autoregulation. The computerized autoregulation equipment graphically demonstrates such changes. However, some patients face much difficulty in learning this simple skill. The absence of a response in their skin temperature—sharply contrasted by the changes seen in other patients during the training sessions—seems to intimidate and discourage them. How might I help such patients overcome this hurdle? I wondered. Rather than being instruments of enlightenment about the inner workings of the human frame, the moving graphs of their biologic functions on the computer screen became obstacles for them. The electrophysiologic sensors were a hindrance—cold, intimidating electronic devices adding to the suffering of the sick. I became increasingly doubtful about the relevance of my work to such patients—the very people who I knew needed self-regulation most.

A MIRACLE IN THE SHOWER

One day it occurred to me that I might try to break the visceral resistance to hand warming by incorporating a simple procedure that the patient can try at home. Patients with strong visceral resistance almost always have cold hands. Could a warm bath or a hot shower help dissipate an individual's visceral resistance? I decided to test the idea.

After standing under a hot shower for several minutes, I remained in the shower, dried myself with a towel, and began my experiment. I let my arms hang loose at my sides and repeated several times the sentence, "My arms and hands are heavy, warm, and loose."

The results of this simple experiment astounded me. My arms and hands flushed to an almost uncomfortable degree. My hands became heavy like lead and throbbed with raw energy. What I expected was a mild hand-warming response—perhaps more pronounced than the responses I was accustomed to with my simple hand-warming exercise. What I did not expect was that my fingertips would throb and pulse so powerfully. I became excited as I recognized how valuable this phenomenon could be in dissolving visceral resistance.

I asked some of my patients to do this simple experiment without telling them about my own experience. Most of them reported exciting responses. The observations of some were identical to mine. Next, I asked a few of them to repeat the experiment and tell me if they succeeded in perceiving clear, strong pulses in their fingertips. Some replied that they already had. Others promised to repeat the experiment and let me know about the results. Most confirmed the perception of unmistakable pulses.

It is one thing for a health professional to ask patients to warm their hands in a laboratory surrounded by complex electromagnetic equipment. It is an altogether different thing for an individual to make a personal discovery of tissue energy in his or her bathroom. That's when I realized how valuable pulses could be for introducing patients to autoregulation. Still, I did not know at that time how important this phenomenon would become to my work.

A SURGEON SENSES HIS HEART RHYTHM

In 1988, at my 25th medical school class reunion, I met Mazhar Jan, M.D., a close friend who practiced general surgery in Milwaukee. He had heard of my interest in self-regulation. We talked about various aspects of this approach to reverse chronic disease and promote health. I asked him if he had ever tried to sense his heart rhythm without feeling for his pulse at the wrists or some other location on his body. To my surprise, he smiled knowingly and said he could, and that he often did, and that he did so without employing any of the autoreg methods that I use with my patients. I asked him how he learned this. He said he just knew he could do it. I wondered how.

Dr. Jan had suffered a heart attack in his early forties. Lying in a bed in an intensive care unit and watching his heart rhythm on a cardiac monitor for interminable hours, an experienced surgeon, no doubt, would have learned how to sense his heart rhythm. So, that is one way of achieving an awareness of one's heart, I mused. But is that the only way one can acquire such awareness of his heart rhythm? I wondered.

Does a person have to suffer from a heart attack to acquire a sensitivity to his heart? Or can he do so by learning some simple method of self-regulation?

The answers to such puzzles usually do not become clear to me immediately. Rather, such puzzles resolve themselves when I least expect it—when driving to and from the office, when accompanying my wife on various errands, or when I am bored by the proceedings of many hospital committee meetings that I am expected to attend.

Was it possible, I wondered, to sense my heart rhythm through some method of self-regulation? The cortical monkey wasn't letting up. I thought of several approaches and tried many, but to no avail. Finally I admitted that clever thinking wasn't going to reveal the answer to that puzzle. My head fixation wasn't enough. Rather, I had to wait for the answer to take form at its own time.

PULSES LEAD TO THE HEART

Exercise speeds up the heart rate. Most people who do not exercise regularly often feel a loud thumping of the heart in the chest during sudden and unexpected bursts of physical activity. A mother dashes after her child, who is running toward a speeding car. After snatching her child, she halts and suffers from heart palpitations.

After my morning limbic ghoraa run, I often do some leg-raising exercises while lying on a carpet. Sometimes this follows a brief period of jumping rope briskly. On one particular day, as I lay down on the carpet, for stretching my back muscles, I could feel my heart beating fast. Rather than let the mind wander, I stayed with and became keenly aware of my heart rhythm. I decided to follow the heart rhythm rather than continue with my usual back exercises. As I expected, my heart rate gradually returned back to normal. But something was different this time. Even though my heart was beating with its normal, regular rhythm, I was still able to clearly sense the heart rhythm. The obvious question was whether it would be possible for me to bring back this awareness without first going through a period of exercise. This is where directed pulses seemed to offer an interesting and clinically useful possibility. What would happen if

I first sensed pulses in my fingertips, then directed them to my heart?

The question raised an exciting prospect. To this end, I did the following simple test: I brought strong pulses to my fingertips with my standard autoreg exercises. I then tried to carry these pulses to the area of my left chest where I had felt the heart rhythm after jumping rope briskly. It worked. I was now able to sense the heart rhythm just as I had after the exercise. (See the latter part of this section for a description of pulse methods.)

Success in autoregulation requires that we abandon our usual competitive, cortical strife for control. It calls for a non-goal-oriented, if-it-happens-it-happens, limbic mode. The core concepts of autoregulation are:

1.   Canceling cortical clutter.
2.   Sensing tissue energy.
3.   Allowing that gentle energy to guide us to a higher healing states.

Autoregulation is not about clever thinking. In fact, the principal hurdle in its path is head-fixation. Chronic thinking leads to an unending recycling of past hurts and precycling of feared, future misery—the two favorites of the cortical monkey. Recycling misery feeds the reverberating cycles of old hurts, long-gone pains, and past memories of sadness.

The discovery that I could perceive my heart activity with self-regulation—the answer to the riddle of heart rhythm—was exciting. The perceptions in a limbic mode had revealed the answer which had eluded the thinking cortical mode for so long.

The next step was simple. I tested this method with many of my patients. With few exceptions, they were able to feel the pulses in their fingertips, then direct them to the heart and perceive the heart rhythms.

TWO CHALAZIA SHRINK AND DISAPPEAR

I developed a chalazion, a type of lump, in the upper eyelid of the right eye. It was the size of one half of a pea. A chalazion is a lump formed by a chronic and intense inflammation of specialized glands in the eyelids. These glands, called meibomian glands, are modified to produce an oily secretion. In chalazia, oily secretions leak out of inflamed glands and form a central cyst. Frequently the inflammatory process results in abscess formation. Sometimes an abscess breaks through the inner membrane of the eyelid and ruptures into the eye. This can have serious consequences. The treatment generally consists of removal of the chalazion by surgery.

Within a few days, a second chalazion appeared close to the first one. The first chalazion grew to the size of a full pea and the second to one half that size. I thought about consulting an ophthalmologist and preparing myself for surgical removal of the chalazia.

I also thought about doing an experiment with directed pulses. I considered the possibility of avoiding surgery by bringing pulses to my eyelids and flushing them with abundant blood. It seemed possible to heal the chalazia with this approach.

All healing occurs with energy. At the level of individual cells in the human body, and at the level of the minute structures within these cells, energy is generated by complex chemical reactions. Nature has designed these reactions to create high energy bonds (called ATP bonds in medical terminology) and to release energy from these bonds in times of need. A disease state represents such a time. All energy reactions require oxygen and micronutrients. Tissues can obtain these elements only through blood. It seemed logical, though simplistic, that chalazia could heal if only I could somehow flush the tissues of the eyelid with blood.

But the surgeon and the pathologist in me raised a warning signal. The inflammation in chalazia causes death of tissues and produces scar tissue. Over the years I have examined hundreds of chalazia under the microscope. I regard this lesion with caution in terms of its ability to destroy healthy tissues.

Could I selectively bring the pulses to one eyelid? Could I effectively sustain such pulses for a long enough period to affect the chalazia? Could mere pulses in the eyelid really clear the pool of oily secretion, arrest inflammation, and prevent scar tissue formation? Would it not be risky to adopt an untried approach to a potentially serious health problem? Even if the pulses could dissolve the chalazia, would they recur? Why not get rid of the chalazia with surgery once and for all?

These were all valid questions. Still, I decided to go ahead with the idea. After all, surgery would always be available to me.

This simple idea turned out to be not only theoretically valid, but both feasible and clinically valuable. It provided me with a firsthand, personal confirmation of the practical value of directed pulses.

By this time, I had become quite proficient at bringing pulses to my fingertips and then directing them to the chest area for sensing my heart rhythm. With the very first attempt, I brought strong pulses to my right eyelid, naturally and effortlessly. Sustaining the pulses in the right eyelid also turned out to be quite an easy task. I brought the pulses to the eyelid by repeating five times each of the following three sentences.

My right upper eyelid is throbbing.
My right upper eyelid is tingling.
My right upper eyelid is pulsating.

After I succeeded in getting strong pulses in the right upper eyelid, I let the pulses go on. Every now and then, when I lost the pulses in the eyelid, I brought them back again by repeating the usual autoreg method for it. I sustained these pulses for over 15 minutes. After a break of several minutes, I brought the pulses back in the right upper eyelid for a second period of about 15 minutes.

The size of a chalazion can be easily measured. One can roll a finger on top of a chalazion pressed against the eyeball and obtain a fairly close measurement of its size. I measured the size of these two chalazia before and after the two periods of pulses in the eyelid. The chalazia shrank to two thirds of their original sizes after application of the pulses.

Hard to believe.
Harder to comprehend.
Hardest of all to accept the utter
simplicity of it.

The temptation to dissolve the two chalazia with more pulses in the eyelid was clear. Instead, I decided to prolong this experiment. I did not practice the method for the pulses in the eyelid for the next three days. The chalazia grew back to their original sizes. At this time, I resumed the pulse methods and practiced four to five times a day, for seven to ten minutes each time. The chalazia shrank to about one fourth their original size in four days.

I decided to continue this experiment for some more time. I stopped the pulse exercise for four days. Once again the chalazia grew back close to their original sizes. I waited three days and started the pulse exercise for the third time. It took me five days to completely clear the chalazia. More than six years have passed, and the chalazia have not recurred.

HIVES, SWOLLEN EYES, STUFFED NOSE, AND AUTOREGULATION

Some time later, I developed a severe food allergy reaction. My left arm developed hives extending from the shoulder to the elbow. My eyes became red, itchy and swollen. My nose became congested. My heart rate quickened and developed palpitations. I reached my office and pulled out adrenaline and Benadryl injections. Reassured by immediate access to these drugs, I decided instead to try the pulses. I reasoned that I could flush the affected tissues with the pulses and eliminate all the chemicals like histamine that cause hives, redness, itching and nasal congestion. Further, the flush of new blood would bring a fresh supply of the enzyme histaminase, and other related enzymes, which the body uses to break down histamine and related chemical compounds.

I directed pulses to my left arm. The hives cleared in about seven minutes. Next, I brought the pulses to my eyes. Some minutes later I felt the itching and swelling around my eyes subside. Next, I focused on my nose.

Research in medicine requires discipline, diligence, perseverance and luck. It is always demanding. Often, it is frustrating. Infrequently, it has its light moments. Bringing the pulses to my nose turned out to be one of those light moments. Strong pulses in my nose converted nasal congestion into a total nasal blockage. No matter how I tried to figure out a way to open my nasal passages with some autoreg method, I drew a blank. That evening I completed my office hours with a totally blocked nose, courtesy of the pulses.

Several months after this incident, I drank some fresh vegetable juice. I didn't realize it included carrots, to which I am allergic. I felt uneasy within a few moments and developed a full-blown allergic reaction with heart palpitations, tightness in the chest, swelling around the eyes and hives. This time, dissolving the allergic reaction with autoreg came readily to me.

This reaction occurred about 15 minutes before I was to attend a meeting of the Medical Executive Committee at Holy Name Hospital. Needless to say, I was on time for the meeting which lasted more than four hours. None of my colleagues suspected that 15 minutes before the meeting I had been in the middle of a severe food allergy reaction. During my days as a physician in the emergency department, I treated such reactions with oxygen, intravenous drip and injections of adrenaline and Benadryl. For patients in my age group, I sometimes hospitalized the patient for extra safety.

I did not need any further proof of the safety and efficacy of autoreg. But some questions remained:

First, would the pulses work for everyone? Second, how many other clinical disorders can be successfully addressed with directed pulses?

FIRST, DO NO HARM

I now started looking in earnest for ways to build upon these observations. Do no harm, first and foremost, is the enduring principle of good medicine. I recognized that beyond my full commitment to the principle of doing no harm were many essential ethical, moral and legal issues that had to be addressed. Informed consent, safety and efficacy, proper research protocols and controls, even the placebo effect, are among the most important issues. But most critical of all was being truthful to myself.

AUTOREGULATION AND HEALING

When a physician teaches self-regulation, the patient, by definition, knows that the physician is not playing the role of healer. The patient knows that healing is a spontaneous phenomenon in injured tissues and that the physician is only facilitating the healing process. Fully aware of the body's ability to heal itself, the patient is now seeking self-regulation, and is willing to be guided by the natural healing energy of the body.

Autoregulation is a path to independence.
Hypnosis and the placebo effect are paths
to dependence on someone else.

Autoregulation fosters healing through self-exploration and self-regulation of one's own biology, but, in order to succeed, the patient must have a full knowledge of his illness. Because the measurable and reproducible electromagnetic responses that accompany healing are clearly visible in the laboratory, issues of informed consent and valid experimental model can be resolved.

Ever mindful of the first principle of good medicine—do no harm—I extended my early personal observations to some selected patients. I focused first on disorders I thought had a reasonable chance of responding to autoregulation with some degree of success. At the very least, I selected cases in which I felt the risks were minimal. I also chose patients who understood the principles of autoregulation, and who I could trust in terms of close follow-up.

ARE PULSES REAL?

Are pulses real, or an imagined response to hypnotic suggestion? Do arteries really throb with pulses, or is it an illusion created by a professional with his clever words?

Many of my patients asked this question during the initial period of autoregulation training. This question is also often raised by professionals who have not experienced such energy responses themselves. Their interest in the subject is purely intellectual and that, of course, is the problem.

During training sessions, I ask everyone in the laboratory to tell me whether or not they felt any energy response. Most individuals say yes, then go on to describe their individual responses. It is not uncommon for some people to feel no energy response during the first couple of exercises. When asked if they think pulses are a real phenomenon, they usually shrug and look askance at the others who said they felt them. In such instances, I make a mental note of that and proceed with subsequent exercises. With rare exception, those who didn't feel pulses in the first exercises do so during subsequent training. When asked the same question about whether pulses are real or not, they grin broadly and nod affirmatively.

The pulses are indeed a real phenomenon. They can be readily monitored with a plethysmograph, an electronic device that measures the range of expansion of tiny blood vessels in the skin. This noninvasive device can be expediently attached to a fingertip with a Velcro band. In my autoregulation lab, I demonstrate to my patients the dynamic moving graph of their pulses on a computer screen.

On the following pages, I illustrate some electro-physiologic patterns that I commonly observe when training patients in the method of directed pulses.

Cortical Mode

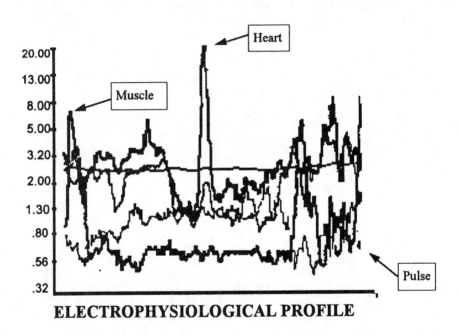

ELECTROPHYSIOLOGICAL PROFILE

This graph shows various body organs in a cortical, stressful mode. The muscle-sensing electrode reveals a very high level of muscle tension and the heart lines shows sharp spikes, indicating distress. The arteries are contracted, indicating poor circulation.

Arteries Are in Spasm,
The Heart Struggles to Cope

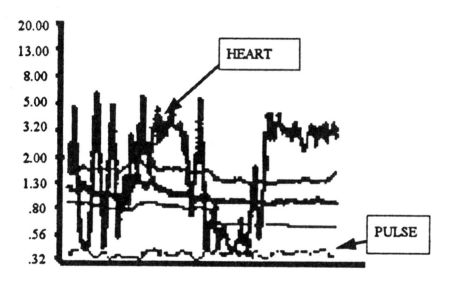

ELECTROPHYSIOLOGICAL PROFILE

In the profile given above, the pulse line produced by the plethysmograph, and indicated by "Pulse," is close to the baseline, indicating very tight arteries. The heart graph, shown by "Heart," displays sharp spikes, indicating how the heart is stressed when it has to pump blood against tightened arteries.

Arteries Open Up,
The Heart Slows Down

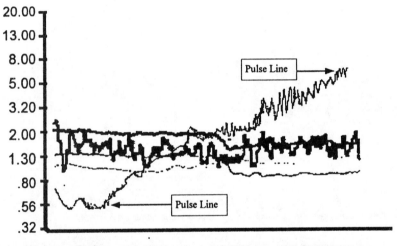

ELECTROPHYSIOLOGICAL PROFILE

The profile shown above demonstrates how the stress on the heart diminishes when the muscle in the arterial wall relaxes and the arteries open up, thus improving the circulation to tissues supplied by the arteries.

The Arteries Open Up,
The Muscles Loosen Up

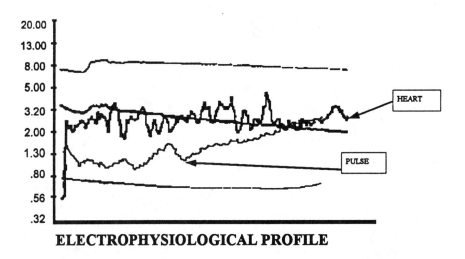

ELECTROPHYSIOLOGICAL PROFILE

The above graph demonstrates how tension in muscles decreases (the two muscle lines gradually slope downward) as arteries open up (the pulse line "Pulse", line climbs up). Note also how the stress on the heart line also diminishes.

Limbic to Cortical Conversion

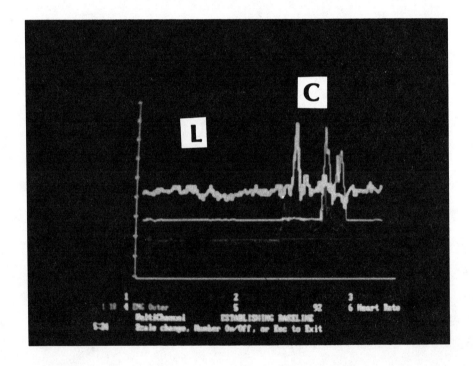

The above graph illustrates a change from a healing, limbic mode to a cortical, disease-causing mode. The limbic-to-cortical transition was recorded about ten seconds after the patient ended autoregulation.

THE WAY WE LOOK AT THE WORLD AROUND US DETERMINES THE STATE OF OUR BIOLOGY

During initial autoregulation training, most of my patients are amazed at the way their biologic profiles change from cortical to limbic modes with autoregulation and back to the cortical mode when they stop autoregulation. These patterns often change instantaneously as the individual moves from a meditating mode to a thinking mode.

It is my practice to guide my patients through 15-minute periods of autoregulation, then stop to explain the various elements of their electrophysiologic profiles. Invariably, during a training session of two and a half to three hours, I am able to demonstrate rather dramatic examples of this phenomenon to my students. The way we look at life around us determines whether we keep our arteries open or closed. All we need to do in the context of autoregulation is to be aware of our tissues and not allow our minds to punish the tissues by closing off the arteries.

TEMPERATURE SHOOTS UP FROM 79 TO 91 DEGREES

Patients with severe environmental sensitivities among civilians, the Gulf War syndrome among veterans, and those suffering a host of autoimmune disorders frequently complain of excessive cold sensitivity—cold hands and feet in common language. I include below some brief comments about this problem. Cold sensitivity is caused by one of the following four mechanisms:

1. Hypothyroidism—underactivity of the thyroid gland—caused by oxidative injury to enzymes involved with thyroid hormone synthesis.
2. Spasm of arteries caused by oxidative stress of adrenergic hypervigilance—excess of stress hormones.
3. Malfunction caused by oxidative injury of the autonomic nervous system that regulate the caliber of arteries.
4. Clumping of blood cells that become sticky—rouleau formation in technical language —caused by oxidative stress on their cell membranes.

Pesticides—organophosphate and chlorinated compounds —and related chemical pollutants are well-recognized for their autonomic receptor toxicity. Damage to such receptors causes spasm of muscles in the wall of blood vessels and leads to vasoconstriction and impaired circulation of tissues, which results in cold hands and feet.

At the Institute, we routinely perform blood tests for an underactive thyroid gland and ask the patient to give us a record of oral and axillary (armpit) temperatures taken before getting out of bed, then three and six hours later. This is followed by appropriate therapies that, in most cases, include a natural thyroid extract. However, repairing injured enzymes and autonomic receptors requires a broad restorative management plan that incorporates the diagnosis and treatment of allergies, nutritional and herbal therapies and training in self-regulation. I discuss this subject at length in *The Canary and Chronic Fatigue.*

Self-regulatory methods that improve circulation are an essential part of any management program for treating cold sensitivity. In my clinical experience, pulses are the best method for this purpose.

It is not uncommon for me to see skin temperatures at the fingertips as low as 77 degrees. (That's where I usually attach sensor electrodes to monitor changes in body temperature during autoregulation.) After years of clinical experience, I can now teach almost all patients with very cold hands how to warm their hands during the first autoregulation session. Indeed, on many occasions I have seen skin temperatures shoot from 77 or 78 degrees to as high as the low 90s in a single session. Such patients are usually very surprised by these dramatic responses. Among their typical reactions:

"I didn't think my hands could get flushed like that."

"If it hadn't happened to me, my God, I would have never believed it!"

"My hands are always freezing. I didn't think this could ever happen to me."

"Who would believe this?"

"Why didn't anyone ever tell me about this? Why did I endure cold hands all those years?"

On some occasions when the hand temperature shoots up, I see patients choke with emotion. Sometimes, they break down and cry.

COLD HANDS, COLD BOWELS, AND BATTERED BOWEL ECOSYSTEMS

It is important to recognize that the biologic stresses we observe in one body organ do not affect that organ alone. Energy patterns in arteries, heart, skin, muscles and other body organs are all interrelated. In fact, a kaleidoscope of biologic inter-relationships is at play. In biology, when we change one thing in one way, we change everything in some way. If stress, depression or injury to autonomic nerve receptors cause spasms of arteries and make a person's hands cold, such a change does not simply affect the arteries in the hands. It affects arteries everywhere to a lesser or greater degree. That person needs to know that not only are the arteries in his hand in spasm, the arteries in his bowel are also in spasm—his bowel is also "cold." A cold bowel is also an oxygen-starved bowel and is a fertile field for various types of yeast that inhabit the bowel ecosystem in health and disease.

Blood sustains life for all tissues. Tissues need a continuous supply of blood rich in oxygen to live, but tight arteries rob tissues of such supply. Hence, there is a shortfall of oxygen and essential nutrients. Since chronic fatigue is a state of accelerated oxidative injury to enzymes and neurotransmitters of the autonomic nervous system, it should come as no surprise that chronically fatigued patients almost always show a pattern of tight arteries. I devote the companion volume, *The Canary and Chronic Fatigue,* to an indepth discussion of the cause, prevention and nondrug management of chronic fatigue.

YEASTS HATE OXYGEN AND FEAST ON SUGAR

Oxygen kills yeasts and sugar feeds them. This is well-established. But how relevant those two facts of biology are to the care of the chronically ill is seldom appreciated by my colleagues. I strongly urge my colleagues who care for the chronically ill not to gloss over this passage. I ask them to take time to study a drop of blood of a patient with cancer, disabling chronic fatigue or other severe autoimmune disorders with a high-resolution microscope equipped with phase-contrast and dark-field optics. I know they will never forget what they see and will never look at chronic illness the same way. As the oxygen in that drop of blood is utilized by red blood cells and the oxygen tension under the cover slip on the microscopic slide diminishes, the yeasts simply blossom. I often examine such slides several hours later and find yeasts assume a hundred creeping, crawling forms, much like the diverse sea life one sees snorkeling. They feed on dying and dead blood cells and their mycotoxins create "microclots" of blood plasma wherever they float. I see such microclots, in smaller amounts and in less dramatic forms, and evidence of cell membrane damage in most fresh blood samples of patients with disrupted bowel ecosystems. I consider such patterns of oxidative injury caused by mycotoxins as one of the core mechanisms of molecular and cellular injury in chronic ecologic and immune disorders as well as in cancer. Where do yeasts in the bloodstream come from? Obviously from the bowel ecosystem. I include here the above brief comments about the role of yeasts and their mycotoxins in the bowel and blood ecosystems to emphasize the need for enhancing blood supply to the bowel with autoregulation. For additional information about such essential ecologic concepts of health and disease, I suggest to the reader relevant chapters in companion volumes *RDA: Rats, Drugs and Assumptions* and *The Canary and Chronic Fatigue.*

A CHOICE

When patients complain of cold hands and feet, I explain to them the relationship between tightened arteries in the hands and feet and those in the bowel, heart, liver and other body organs. Then I give them a choice:

They can keep their arteries tight, rob their organs of energy, and stress their biology.

Or,

they can keep their arteries open, nourish their organs with nutrients and energy, be kind to their biology, and stay healthy.

During initial training, it is sometimes useful to give patients pictures of their biologic profiles, showing points of stress and how they are relieved by autoregulation. Such pictures provide a method of directed imagery. However, once an individual learns the basic methods of autoregulation, directed imagery in my experience is not only unnecessary, it indeed interferes with reaching higher states of healing energy. Notwithstanding its early and rather limited advantages, directed imagery is still a cortical device and best avoided after the initial stages of autoregulation.

PULSES BECOME A REGULAR PART OF OUR INSTITUTE VOCABULARY

Within a year after beginning my work with autoregulation, pulses became a regular part of our vocabulary. This simple word allows us to talk freely about the basic concept, training and practice of autoregulation. I include some examples below:

Kathy, a 57-year-old college professor with a chronic, unrelenting headache, spoke the following words during a visit four weeks after her initial training in the methods of autoreg:

"I brought the pulses to my fingertips and felt something like a bubble burst in my temple areas. Then, suddenly, my headache was gone."

For many years, Doris, a 53-year-old woman, had been on Synthroid (a synthetic form of thyroid hormone) for an underactive thyroid gland. Over the years, her attempts to discontinue the drug's use or reduce the dose had resulted in a recurrence of the symptoms. She consulted me to see if we could use the autoregulation approach to help her discontinue the drug therapy, or at least cut back the dosage.

I instructed her in autoregulation, taught her how to direct pulses to her thyroid gland, then reduced the dose of her thyroid replacement medication by one half. Such patients often suffer symptoms such as loss of vigor, tiredness, irritability and weight gain when the thyroid replacement hormone is withheld. I cautioned her to increase the drug dosage if any of these symptoms developed. I didn't know how the thyroid would react to the increased blood supply brought on by autoregulation. She called me several weeks later and reported:

"I have reduced the dose of the thyroid hormone by one half as you recommended. I have had no symptom recurrence this time as I did on previous occasions. By the way, I have no trouble with pulses in my thyroid gland. I bring them on five or six times a day."

Stephanie, a woman in her early sixties, suffered from intermittent claudication—painful muscle spasms in the legs caused by arteriosclerosis (hardening of the arteries) that also clogs the vessel lumen. Robbed of their blood, oxygen, and energy, muscles go into spasms that cause intense pain.

Here is what Stephanie told me during a follow-up visit several weeks later:

"I woke up with the sharp pain of a cramp in my leg. I could not remember the steps of autoreg you taught me. I was very confused. So I just yelled, 'tingle, legs, tingle.' My pain subsided. I went back to sleep."

Here are quotes from some other patients:

> *"When you started the class, I had a lot of
> stiffness and some pain in my neck. Now it
> is gone."*

> *"I wanted to cancel this class. I've had this
> intestinal virus and didn't know if I could
> go through the class without running off to
> the bathroom every 20 minutes. But
> nothing has happened during the last three
> hours."*

> *"My sinuses have cleared up. Amazing! I
> still had a wheeze from my asthma attack
> when we started. Now I breathe much
> easier."*

> *"Skin itching is gone."*

> *"Relaxed! Very relaxed! I had a tough day.
> I was very tense. Now I'm relaxed."*

AUTOREGULATION STOPS COUGH

In the summer of 1995, Carol Grieden-Burger, Director of
Nursing at our Institute, began teaching autoregulation at the

Institute. One day, she and I were preparing for a class. A patient coughed incessantly. Carol became very concerned that her cough would distract everyone. I suggested to Carol that we might give her our Throat Protocol, a vitamin gargle formula that works well for such problems, to soothe her throat and reduce cough. As Carol stood up to fetch the gargle formula, I wondered what would happen if we tried to soothe her cough reflex by eliminating the stress on it with autoregulation. "Carol, let's wait. Let's see what autoregulation can do for her," I said, half jokingly, not knowing what to expect. She gave me a quizzical look, then smiled and proceeded with her instruction.

That autoregulation class lasted for about three hours. The patient troubled by the incessant cough hardly ever coughed when we did various autoregulation exercises, but did so whenever we stopped to explain to the group their biologic profiles on the video screen. Everyone in the laboratory was pleasantly surprised—and evidently amused—by what they saw. The next day, I asked Carol what she thought of the incident. "I was shocked!" she grinned broadly as she spoke in her Swiss accent.

REINS ON PULSES

Normally the walls of arteries in our body are held in a state of partial contraction. In medical terminology, this is called vascular tone. It is regarded as the peripheral resistance that is essential for maintaining pressure inside these blood vessels. This is a precise scientific definition of the term "blood pressure."

The state of partial contraction of the arterial wall is maintained by electromagnetic impulses generated in a small area in the lower part of the brain called the vasomotor center. These impulses travel along specialized nerves called sympathetic and parasympathetic nerve fibers. These nerves, along with their relay stations (autonomic ganglia), have been given the name autonomic nervous system.

TAKING THE FOOT OFF THE BRAKE PEDAL

Some very anxious patients tense up visibly when I begin instruction in simple methods of autoregulation. The simple act of closing their eyes raises their stress level. That sometimes reminds me of my first driving lesson.

My father had a tiny British-built Morris 8 model car, which was driven by his driver (a colonial expression for chauffeur). We had a long oval driveway in front of the government bungalow where we lived in the city of Multan. In the afternoon when my father would return from his court, my brothers and I would ask the driver for a ride in the car and to let us control the steering wheel of the car as he controlled the gas and brake pedals. I was barely thirteen. After some time, I became good at steering. Then one day I persuaded the driver to let me operate the whole thing, the gas and brake pedals, the clutch and, of course, the steering wheel. I never forgot the first spine-jolting experience the car gave me. As I took my foot off the brake pedal, the car simply took off (at least that's the way it seemed to me then). Rather than gently apply the brakes, in utter confusion I slammed my foot on the gas pedal, then abruptly turned the steering wheel. A thick hedge of strong bushes stopped the car. My whole body shook for a while.

The stress of life works our bodies in a somewhat similar way. Many people exist in an overdrive mode. It is hard for them to simply ease off the brake pedals and gently put their foot on the gas pedal. They keep their muscles taut, eyes strained, hearts pumped up, and lungs hyperventilating. For them, anything that attempts to shift their state of hypervigilance to an even, calm mode exaggerates the stress. This is the simple and—in my view—the only valid explanation of events that take place when people move from a noisy, overdrive state to limbic silence. Silence for them is insufferable. Earlier in my work with self-regulation, I lost some patients for this reason. Now I take time to explain such aspects of autoregulation before I begin instruction and prepare them for the initial turbulence.

CORTICAL DEBRAKING

"Cortical debraking" is a term I sometimes use to explain to my patients the nature of initial visceral resistance to autoregulation.

Typically, a patient becomes uncomfortable as he closes his eyes to begin autoregulation. He may feel constriction in his chest. He may feel tightness in his abdomen. If he is reclining in a chair, he may suddenly sit up with evident distress. I have seen patients suddenly become tense just as they were beginning to feel their muscles become limp, loose and limbic. In most instances, they are able to proceed with autoreg and overcome the initial visceral resistance.

The idea of using this term "cortical debraking" came to me once as I watched a patient begin to relax, then jolt with obvious discomfort. It was as if she slammed her foot on her *cortical brakes* with full force just as she was beginning to ease her foot off it, much like a teenager taking his first driving lesson. A student driver requires patience and practice to become good at gently taking his foot off the brake pedal so his car can roll forward smoothly and without any jolts. It is the same way with cortical debraking. A sudden release can be jolting. A beginner needs patience and practice with autoreg.

Most of the time, such cortical debraking—negative energy responses—are of mild degree and of short duration. Uncommonly, such responses can be extremely troublesome and require persistent efforts. I discuss this subject at length and describe some specific examples of such phenomenon in the chapter, The Bite of the Gray Dog.

FINGERTIPS TO FINGERTIPS PULSES

I focus on the fingertips during early training in autoreg for a simple reason. Fingertips contain the richest supply of sympathetic nerve fibers. It is easy to see the wisdom of Nature in this. We use our fingertips for more functions than any other body organ. It also means that the walls of arteries in our fingertips have the tightest reins on them from the vasomotor center in the brain. It also explains why our fingers and hands are the first body organs to feel cold when we are stressed or become depressed.

There is yet another simple method that many of my patients found to be very useful during early training. This method is especially valuable for those who do succeed in getting the pulses when training with a professional but are unable to get them on their own.

In this method, I ask my patients to hold their hands together in their laps with the fingertips of one hand touching the fingertips of the other. Juxtaposition of the fingertips assists in the perception of the pulses. Again, once a person succeeds in getting the pulses, he should separate his two hands to see if he can sustain the pulses when his fingertips are not touching.

Children learn autoregulation fast. They can be quickly taught to ease up on these autonomic reins on their arteries and let the pulses flow freely.

PULSES IN THE WASHBASIN

I wrote earlier that a vast majority of patients in my autoregulation class learn the method of directed pulses during the very first training session. It was different when I began teaching autoregulation to my patients over ten years ago. At that time, many patients were frustrated by their inability to perceive any energy in their tissues with autoregulation. This was quite common among very ill patients. Even when some of them felt the pulses during my autoregulation class, they were unable to perceive or sustain pulses later when they tried the method on their own. It didn't take long before their angst became my frustration. I began to think of ways that I could help such patients overcome their systemic resistance.

The answer to the riddle became obvious one day in my laboratory when a woman in her mid-eighties related her experience. She had patiently sat through the training session for more than two hours without perceiving any energy in her hands as other patients in the class related their positive experiences. After the last autoregulation exercise, suddenly her face beamed with excitement as she loudly proclaimed that finally she had felt the pulses. Then she added, "I guess it happened now because my hands have been slowly and steadily warming during the class, even though I didn't feel clear pulses."

Like a flash, her comment gave me the idea of using warm water for the initial warming of hands, before beginning autoregulation. The next question was simple and predictable: What would be the simplest and most convenient way to warm hands?

In the method of pulses in the washbasin, a person dips both hands in a washbasin full of lukewarm water for five to ten minutes. When the temperature of the hands and fingers rises to that of the warm water, the person takes his hands out of the washbasin, dries them and begins autoregulation.

I have now validated the clinical efficacy of this method with extensive experience. Most patients who report initial difficulties with autoregulation find this method very useful in breaking the initial systemic resistance.

Pulses in the washbasin may be tried in a kitchen or bathroom sink or in a warm-water bathtub.

PULSES IN THE SHOWER

As I stated earlier, pulses in the shower is another method I tried—and found to be very effective—during my early years of research with autoregulation. I experimented with this method before I thought of using warm water in a washbasin for overcoming initial systemic resistance. This was an important discovery for me—a powerful demonstration of the phenomena of energy in self-regulation work. I moved on to the method of pulses in the washbasin for some important reasons, which I describe later in this section.

I strongly caution chronically ill persons against this exercise. Specifically, those with high blood pressure and heart disease must not attempt this method. Furthermore, all readers must read about the three cautions given on the following pages before trying this simple method.

Persons in robust health may try this method as follows: After a relaxing bath or shower, dry yourself with a towel. Stand upright and still for a few moments. Keep your back and neck straight and loose. Now move your shoulders a little and feel your arms literally hang loose from your shoulders. Shift your awareness to your hands. (Do not try to focus or concentrate on your hands or on anything. Also, do not try to *unfocus,* since that is also a cortical trap.) Simply be aware of your hands, keeping them limp and loose. Now repeat to yourself seven times each of the following five sentences:

- My hands are heavy and warm.
- My hands are heavy and warm and limp and loose.
- My fingertips are tingling.
- My fingertips are throbbing.
- My fingertips are pulsating.

At the end of this simple exercise, in all likelihood your hands will feel heavy like lead and very comfortable. You will probably also feel clear and strong pulses in most, if not all, ten fingertips. On rare occasions, extremely ill patients have told me they did not succeed in feeling the pulses with their first attempt. Such people require more than one trial.

After you have succeeded in getting the pulses, you may continue this exercise for as long as you wish. If you lose the pulses, you can easily bring them back by repeating the same sentences.

WHEN NOT TO DO PULSES IN THE SHOWER

For emphasis, I reiterate that the method of pulses in the shower should not be tried under certain circumstances. There are three important considerations.

First,

> Read the paragraphs on cortical braking on the previous pages. You may be surprised or even overwhelmed by the way tissues respond. Pulses are an element of self-discovery and it is a very pleasant surprise. Still, it is necessary to be prepared to receive the response from your tissues.

Second,

> If you are under treatment by your physician for a specific disease, please check with him or her. It may be necessary to practice the initial training under professional supervision. Autoregulation is regulating yourself. But in the midst of an established illness, it is necessary to be cautious.

Third,

> There are other more suitable methods for ill patients to begin practicing autoregulation methods. One good alternative is pulses in the washbasin.

WHEN NOT TO DO PULSES

Directed pulses are a simple, safe, and useful method for stress control and for increasing the blood supply (and healing energy) to any part of the body. In general, one cannot overdo the pulses. I have taught this technique to a very large number of patients. There are, however, a few situations where it is best to avoid directing pulses to some part of the body.

1. The pain in acutely inflamed tissues may be intensified with the dilatation of blood vessels brought about with pulses. The same holds for acute abscesses where the pulses may precipitate throbbing pain.

2. Congestion in the nose and sinuses is usually made worse with the pulses.

3. An established severe headache is generally made worse with this method. The pulses are useful for dissolving headaches, but only during the initial period.

4. While internal wounds heal, dilated vessels carry the risk of internal bleeding. A patient underwent prostatectomy. The wound in his bladder stopped bleeding in two days. He was very proficient in the method of the pulses. On the third day, without consulting with me, he tried it on his own to facilitate wound healing by sending the pulses to his gland. Within an hour, the wound started bleeding. He called me for advice. I told him not to do the pulses. He stopped and, within a few hours, the bleeding stopped.

AUTONOMIC AND SOMATIC NERVOUS SYSTEMS

The nervous system in the human body—I was taught in medical school—comprises two distinct and discrete systems: a somatic nervous system that is under our voluntary control and an autonomic nervous system that is beyond our control. When we lift a glass of water, we willfully use muscles in an arm. This is an example of the functioning of the somatic nervous system—the thinking mind directs activity in muscles. When a person's blood pressure rises due to tightness in his arteries and he tries to order his tightened arteries to loosen up, nothing happens. (If the thinking mind was capable of such a feat, none of us physicians would ever take drugs for high blood pressure.) That is an example of autonomic function—a bodily function that is outside the reach of the thinking mind.

All our prevailing medical ideas of the function of the heart rate and rhythm, arterial tone, and electromagnetic energy in skin and muscles are based on this fundamental distinction between somatic and autonomic nervous systems. And so are ideas concerning the treatment of diseases affecting these organs.

Earlier work with biofeedback research led many investigators to conclude that autonomic nervous functions were also under voluntary control. The evidence for this viewpoint was derived from changes observed during biofeedback in heart rate, blood pressure, brain wave patterns and a host of other autonomic functions. This led to the widespread—and, in my view, mistaken—belief that mind-over-body healing works and that the thinking mind can learn to control the function of the heart, arteries, bowel and other body organs previously thought to be outside its reach. This erroneous belief also spawned the now thriving mind-over-body industry.

The distinction between the somatic (voluntary) and autonomic (involuntary) nervous systems is the primary reason why mainstream physicians do not put much stock in the mind-over-body healing notions espoused by the New Age gurus and so heartily accepted by the general public. On this issue I stand firmly among my colleagues in the mainstream. The thinking mind does not—it cannot—heal the injured tissues. How can it? How can the thinking mind direct the healing phenomenon in injured tissues when it does not even understand it? To date, I have never met a person who claims to understand how healing occurs. Specifically, how does an injured cell know it is injured? How does a cell know its neighbor cell has died, so it must multiply to fill the void left by the dead cell? And how do multiplying cells know when there are enough of them and they can cease replicating? A cell is a cosmos. Within it lie myriads of organelles. How do the organelles on one side of the cell know those on the other side have been zapped by radiotherapy or chemotherapy? When a child is hit by a car and loses a lot of blood, the cells in his bone marrow multiply rapidly to make up for the blood loss. How do the parent cells sitting smugly in the bone marrow know their offspring cells have been lost through gaping wounds in the skin?

One can ask such questions endlessly. Pathologists like me who have studied injured cells and tissues with microscopes for decades know there are no easy answers to any of those questions. The thinking mind simply does not know the answers. And yet, the gurus of mind-over-body healing continue to incubate grand schemes for using the mind to ordain healing in injured tissues.

I do not believe the thinking mind can ever heal injured tissues. In the same vein, to date I have never seen any evidence that the thinking mind can normalize raised blood pressure or slow the heart rate. These functions of the autonomic nervous system are manifestly outside the domain of the thinking mind. I address this subject in greater detail in the companion volume, *RDA: Rats, Drugs and Assumptions*.

Artists, musicians, and poets usually find the principles of autoregulation—autonomic training with energy dynamics—simple to understand and its practice easy to follow. I suppose it is because they are comfortable with abstract notions of life and energy. This group usually progresses rapidly, and I am able to see objective, electrophysiologic evidence of this progress during the very first training session. Lawyers and accountants often have more difficulty in the initial stages. Physicians often find autoregulation tedious, as do nurses to a lesser degree.

AUTOREGULATION ISN'T MIND-OVER-BODY HEALING, IT'S THE EXACT OPPOSITE

In my view the core belief of the biofeedback community that individuals can be trained to bring involuntary autonomic nervous functions under voluntary control of the thinking mind is erroneous.

So then, how does one reconcile the commonly observed phenomena of "mind-over-body" control of asthma, colitis, and PMS with the clear inability of the thinking mind to understand the healing response in injured tissues, let alone direct it with volition? The answer to that question is really quite simple: In self-regulation, the mind does not do any healing. Rather, when it is excluded—canceled out with any method—the body slips into its natural state of healing energy. Thus, healing in self-regulation isn't a mind-over-body phenomenon, it's the exact opposite.

I address this subject in more than one place in this volume because I see it as the single most important obstacle in the path of healing among my patients.

> *Healing occurs when we are unfocused.*
> *Energy events that bring about healing in*
> *injured tissues are facilitated when we*
> *escape the tyranny of the thinking mind.*

I measure the results of such training sessions with accurate, objective, and reproducible electromagnetic technology. It is quite rare for me to see a patient who fails in this completely. Needless to say, some people learn much faster than others. At times, the progress of patients in the throes of intense chronic suffering is slow.

AUTOREGULATION FOR SKIN CANCER

I will give one more example. This is not an actual case history, but it will allow me to make an essential point.

A patient consults me for a skin tumor. I recommend a biopsy that reveals a basal cell carcinoma. A basal cell carcinoma is a meek cancer. It grows slowly. It takes months and years to invade the underlying tissues. It almost never metastasizes (spreads to distant organs). Now, suppose this patient previously had learned autoregulation for some other disease such as asthma. He had been successful in controlling asthma attacks with autoreg methods (without drugs but with nutritional support and allergy treatment). He is well-versed with the principles and practices of autoregulation. I will give him the option of healing his skin cancer with autoreg methods. I know this method will not be a very difficult task for him. Both he and I can easily keep a close watch on his skin cancer.

Next, let us consider a different setting. The biopsy discloses a melanoma. A melanoma is a rabid, highly malignant tumor that shows no respect for body tissues. It can invade the blood and lymphatic vessels within weeks to months, spread to lungs and other body organs, and prove fatal. In this case I will insist that the patient have the tumor removed by surgery without any delay. Only after that will I support the patient's request for use of autoreg methods to enhance immunity and reduce the chance of tumor recurrence.

I relate here another case history. A woman in her mid-fifties consulted me for breast cancer that had spread to lymph glands in her axillae, lungs and bones. Her breast cancer was a small lump when it was diagnosed with a biopsy about three years earlier. Small-sized cancer of the breast—less than one half inch in diameter—when not associated with node involvement can be cured by a simple surgical removal in over ninety percent of women. Her physician had recommended surgical removal of the tumor, which she had forcefully declined. She visited me to see if I could add something to her comprehensive program for control of cancer comprised of herbs, vitamins, coffee enemas, exercise and meditation. Evidently, her program of natural therapies had not worked. (No therapies work in *all* cases.) I reviewed the whole case, made some recommendations, and suggested she might spend several hours with me during autoregulation classes. She thanked me, stood up, and walked to the door. There she stopped, hesitated for several moments, then turned and asked, "Dr. Ali, do you think I made a mistake in turning down surgery when the cancer was very small?" I felt the anguish in her words, wondered how I could mitigate it, then decided to reply in simple words. "Yes, in my view, that was an error."

Making the right choice when facing therapies for cancer is always a very hard decision. There is no simple way out. I discuss this subject at length in the companion volume *The Crab and the Other Side of Cancer.*

FOUND AND PROFOUND

In self-regulation, meditation and spiritual work, the experience of others can be an interesting topic for conversation at the dinner table, but it is never truly enlightening. There is seldom anything profound in such conversations. Autoregulation, I write earlier, is a process by which one enters a healing energy state. When in such a state, all intellectual function ceases. There are no perceptions except those of energy. There are no clever healing words. There are no mind-over-body schemes. There is no point to any conversation.

Many people find easy relief of symptoms in hypnosis. That is desirable. However, in my experience such symptom relief rarely lasts long. There are no profound insights in hypnosis.

Received wisdom is of limited value in autoregulation and other similar energy states. There are paths to self discovery at deeper, visceral energy levels. The healing energy I refer to in this context is in the domain of the invisible. It is about linkage with the larger *presence* that permeates and surrounds each of us at all times. *That is the source of all healing.* One needs to understand fully that there is nothing profound in the words that I use in autoregulation training to the beginner. Words help only in canceling the cortical clutter. Nor do I believe there can be anything profound in the words that someone else might propose for preparing to enter the healing energy state. In essence, autoregulation is about spirituality. What is found easily in life is rarely profound. Perhaps nowhere else is that truer than in the case of healing and spiritual work.

ANGER AND PULSES

Anger is a major risk factor for disease. Angry people do not heal well.

Jane, a 30-year-old schoolteacher, consulted me for chronic joint pains, bowel cramps with flatulence, sinus allergy, and chronic fatigue. What she did not include in her complaints, but was quite evident during her first visit, was an anger that permeated her whole being. By the second visit, some of Jane's anger was directed at me. By her third visit, I began to have serious reservations about my ability to help. But autoreg and allergy and nutritional protocols did work and gave Jane considerable relief. Slowly, over a period of months, Jane mellowed and I didn't see the fury of anger beneath the words she used during the visit. She began to relate her experiences with autoregulation, especially the benefits of minute-reg. One day during a follow-up visit, she spoke the following words:

"You know, I don't get angry at my students anymore, and I don't curse the drivers ahead of me on the road."

Heavy loads of tension and anger are common among patients who have suffered for years, whose conventional laboratory tests have been negative, and who have been told they have all-in-the-head problems. Such patients do not get better until they learn to extinguish the oxidative fireworks under their skin. I discuss this subject in the companion volume *What Do Lions Know About Stress?*

Exercises for the Pulses

The following is the text of the autoreg tape I use for my patients. You may wish to use this text to prepare a tape for your own use in your own voice. I encourage my patients to do so. I also encourage them to add to this text additional material which they may find suitable. For the beginner, I recommend my own tapes (available from the Institute, (201) 586-4111).

This text for my tapes is copyrighted material and may not be used to prepare tapes for sale or distribution to others in other ways.

In autoregulation, words are not important; the energy responses to which they lead are. Words are used only to cancel the cortical clutter and escape into limbic openness. The gentle guiding energy knows how to direct itself to the parts of the body under duress.

The tone of the voice, the emphasis on certain words, the spacing between successive sentences, and intervals between the various steps of this autoregulation exercise enhance its clinical benefits. The reader may begin autoregulation with my tapes, suitable tapes prepared by other professionals, or make his own tapes using the text that follows. Again, the core idea of autoregulation is to enter a healing energy state. It matters little what particular words, phrases, or sentences can help an individual to enter the healing energy state that I describe in this volume.

In the tape text that follows, I take the beginner through some simple but effective steps that I have found to be useful after extensive clinical experience. This tape is for initial training in autoregulation. Our objectives at this stage are to learn how to be aware of our patterns of circulation, our breathing cycles, and the electromagnetic energy in our skin, muscles and other tissues. These basic skills are essential for success in advanced methods of attending to different parts of our biology with autoregulation. It is important for the reader to practice basic autoregulation methods before seeking higher energy states that are only possible with deep *methodless* spiritual work.

PULSES WITH AUTOREGULATION TAPE

Assume the comfortable position you were in when we did autoreg in the lab together. You are sitting comfortably, at the edge of the chair. Your back is straight, maintaining the natural forward curve. Your knees are about 12 inches apart. Your feet are flat on the floor. Your hands are resting on your thighs, your palms facing upward. Your eyes are closed. Move your shoulders gently and let the muscles settle in so you feel your arms hanging loose and free from your shoulders. If you wish to change your position to make yourself more comfortable during autoregulation training, please feel free to do so. The position I describe is the ideal position for most people who practice autoreg.

As we begin autoreg, our cortical mind rebels. It asserts itself in many ways. It will wander off. When that happens, we will let it do so. We will not fight it. We will stay with the autoreg steps. Our cortical mind will begin to judge and censor us. We will let it do so. If it distracts us with angry thoughts, we will let it do so. If it brings us images of past hurts, we will let it do so. We will stay with the autoreg steps. If it argues with us and tells us autoregulation will not work, we will let it do so. We will stay with the autoregulation steps.

After the initial instruction, I give my patients a tape that I specifically prepare for this purpose. (This tape is available from the Institute.) With practice, most people can learn, within days or weeks, how to do the pulses without any external help from a tape or a professional. Patients with severe chronic ailments, as I mentioned earlier, usually require extended training with a professional.

Together we will free limbic healing energy from the captivity of the thinking cortical mind.

****

Breathe in and feel your stomach gently roll out.
Breathe out and feel your stomach gently roll back in.
Breathe in and feel your stomach gently roll out.
Breathe out and feel your stomach gently roll back in.
Breathe in and feel your stomach gently roll out.
Breathe out and feel your stomach gently roll back in.
Breathe in and feel your stomach gently roll out.
Breathe out and feel your stomach gently roll back in.

My hands are heavy and warm.
My hands are heavy and warm.
My hands are heavy and warm and limp.
My hands are heavy and warm and limp.
My hands are heavy and warm and limp and loose.
My hands are heavy and warm and limp and loose.
My hands are heavy and warm and limp and loose.

                    ****

My feet are heavy and warm.
My feet are heavy and warm.
My feet are heavy and warm and limp.
My feet are heavy and warm and limp.
My feet are heavy and warm and limp and loose.
My feet are heavy and warm and limp and loose.
My feet are heavy and warm and limp and loose.

                    ****

My hands and feet are heavy and warm and
    limp and loose.
My hands and feet are heavy and warm and
    limp and loose.
My hands and feet are heavy and warm and
    limp and loose.
My hands and feet are heavy and warm and
    limp and loose.
My hands and feet are heavy and warm and

limp and loose.
My hands and feet are heavy and warm and
limp and loose.
My hands and feet are heavy and warm and
limp and loose.

****

My leg muscles are heavy and warm and limp and loose.
My leg muscles are heavy and warm and limp and loose.
My leg muscles are heavy and warm and limp and loose.
My leg muscles are heavy and warm and limp and loose.
My leg muscles are heavy and warm and limp and loose.
My leg muscles are heavy and warm and limp and loose.
My leg muscles are heavy and warm and limp and loose.

****

My thigh muscles are heavy and warm and limp and loose.
My thigh muscles are heavy and warm and limp and loose.
My thigh muscles are heavy and warm and limp and loose.
My thigh muscles are heavy and warm and limp and loose.
My thigh muscles are heavy and warm and limp and loose.
My thigh muscles are heavy and warm and limp and loose.
My thigh muscles are heavy and warm and limp and loose.

My shoulder and neck muscles are limp and loose.
My shoulder and neck muscles are limp and loose.
My shoulder and neck muscles are limp and loose.

I am on a beach. It is a clear day. The sky is deep blue. The breeze is soft and gentle on my face. I see the waves breaking on the white sand. I see gulls floating on the water. The breeze is soft and gentle on my face. I see the waves breaking on white sand.

I see water waves breaking on the white sand.
I see water waves breaking on the white sand.
I see water waves breaking on the white sand.
I see water waves breaking on the white sand.
I see water waves breaking on the white sand.
I see water waves breaking on the white sand.
I see water waves breaking on the white sand.
I see water waves breaking on the white sand.

****

I see seagulls floating in the air.
I see seagulls floating in the air.
I see seagulls floating in the air.
I see seagulls floating in the air.
I see seagulls floating in the air.
I see seagulls floating in the air.
I see seagulls floating in the air.
I see seagulls floating in the air.

****

I see water waves breaking on the white sand.

I see water waves breaking on the white sand.
I see water waves breaking on the white sand.
I see water waves breaking on the white sand.
I see water waves breaking on the white sand.
I see water waves breaking on the white sand.
I see water waves breaking on the white sand.
I see water waves breaking on the white sand.

****

My hands are heavy like lead, and limp and loose.
My hands are heavy like lead, and limp and loose.
My hands are heavy like lead, and limp and loose.
My hands are heavy like lead, and limp and loose.
My hands are heavy like lead, and limp and loose.
My hands are heavy like lead, and limp and loose.
My hands are heavy like lead, and limp and loose.
My hands are heavy like lead, and limp and loose.

****

My fingertips are throbbing.
All ten of my fingertips are throbbing.
All ten of my fingertips are throbbing.
All ten of my fingertips are throbbing.

My fingertips are tingling.
All ten of my fingertips are tingling.
All ten of my fingertips are tingling.

All ten of my fingertips are tingling.

My fingertips are pulsating.
All ten of my fingertips are pulsating.
All ten of my fingertips are pulsating.
All ten of my fingertips are pulsating.

My toes are throbbing.
My toes are throbbing.
My toes are throbbing.

****

I can imagine the space in the back of my throat.
I feel the space in the back of my throat expand when I
    breathe in.
I feel the space in the back of my throat expand when I
    breathe in.
I feel the space in the back of my throat expand when I
    breathe in.

I can imagine the volume of my right hand.
I can feel my hand swell up as I breathe in.
I can feel my hand swell up as I breathe in.
I can feel my hand swell up as I breathe in.

I feel energy in my right hand.
I feel energy in my right hand.
I feel energy in my right hand.

I feel energy in both my hands.

I feel energy in both my hands.
I feel energy in both my hands.

I feel energy in my hands and feet.
I feel energy in my hands and feet.
I feel energy in my hands and feet.

I feel energy in all parts of my body.
I feel energy in all parts of my body.
I feel energy in all parts of my body.

****

I will now count to three, and this will end the autoreg session. If you feel that your body tissues are loose and limp and limbic and wish to stay that way, please do so. You may end autoreg at a later time when that feels right to you.

Three--two--one.
You may gently open your eyes.
Gently stretch your fingers and toes.
Sit comfortably for a few moments. Then you may slowly rise. Practice minute-reg as often as you can during the day while doing your day's work.

SCANNING THE BODY

Sensing tissue energy is an essential element in all types of self-regulation with energy. Autoregulation is no exception. Just as a person can sense warmth in hands or pulses in fingertips with simple self-suggestive sentences, it is possible to sense energy of other tissues with a similar approach. Sensing is then followed by "staying with the energy" in the tissues or body organ in question.

Talat, my wife, uses the expression "scan the body, then respond to what needs responding." It is a succinct description of a method that she has used extensively for herself and for her students. She recommends the following simple steps:

1. Scan the whole body for unease, discomfort or pain—moving slowly from hands, arms, shoulders, neck, head, face, torso and limbs.

2. Isolate tissues under duress—keep your awareness fixed to those tissues.

3. Sense the energy or absence of it in the tissues that are the focus of your awareness.

4. Breathe into—or into and through—the tissues under duress. A simple method for this is to repeat any of the following sentences several times until one begins to sense an energy response in that particular tissue:

4.1   I breathe in and my right hand swells up with energy.

4.2   I breathe in and feel both hands swell up with energy.

4.3   I breathe in and feel my eyes swell up with energy.

4.4   I breathe in and my right thigh swells up with energy.

4.5   I breathe in and feel my back muscles swell up with energy.

4.6   I breathe in and feel my abdomen swell up with energy.

Some reader may raise an obvious question here: Aren't these examples of mind-over-body healing? On a superficial level, yes they are. But as I discuss in many parts of this volume, these are in reality examples of giving the cortical monkey a taste of his own medicine. By breathing into or through a tissue under duress, what we really achieve is stillness in the mind. We exclude the mind from our state. Or, to be more precise, we use breathing methods to break the chains of the cortical clutter. Once we perceive the tissue energy, we are guided by the gentle limbic healing energy.

What is freedom? To the extent that human beings can be free, it is the freedom from the need to be free that sets us free. To the extent that we can feel secure, it is the recognition that there can be no complete security in life. Thus, freedom and security are the gifts we receive when we learn to trust that larger presence that surrounds and permeates each of us at all times.

What Do Lions Know About Stress?

Chapter 5

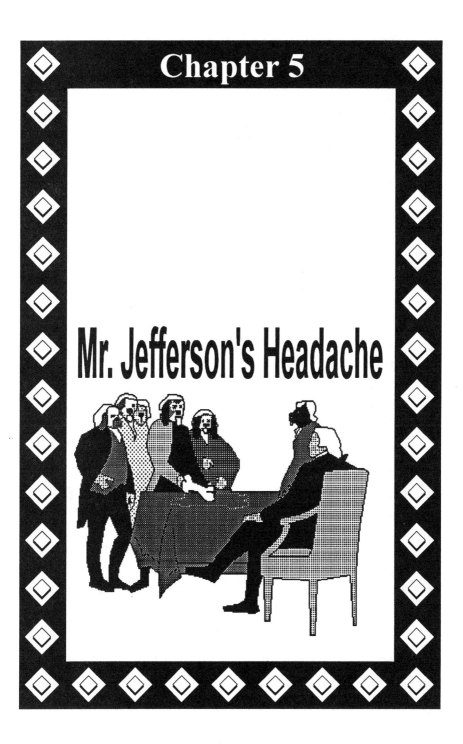

Mr. Jefferson's Headache

Some personal experiences and observations have profoundly influenced my thinking about sickness, self-regulation and healing. Many of such experiences played a direct role in the evolution of my concepts of the principles and practice of autoregulation. Below, I briefly describe some of those experiences.

MY MIGRAINE HEADACHE ATTACKS

I suffered migraine headache attacks from the time of my childhood until the age of 47, when I learned to dissolve them with autoregulation. My migraine attacks were fairly consistent in pattern. The attacks began with a sense of heaviness in my head. Within an hour or so, the heaviness would turn into a dull headache felt all over. Some time later, the headache localized to my forehead and temple regions and progressively worsened until it caused eye discomfort and nausea. An hour or so later, nausea culminated in projectile vomiting. Eventually the headache became severe, unrelenting and disabling. Oral painkillers never helped since the pills always returned with vomitus. Finally, I would inject myself with Demerol (a potent narcotic and powerfully addictive drug) to obtain some relief. Demerol usually increased my vomiting until I would doze off for several hours. On the day after the injection, I usually felt lethargic and hated the effects of the injection.

I suffered such migraine headache attacks all through my years of high school, college and medical school in Pakistan; emergency medicine and surgical training in England; pathology residency and practice of surgical and clinical pathology in the

United States. During this time, I taught at medical and dental schools. Yet, no one ever mentioned to me that there may indeed be an end to my periods of misery with simple work with self-regulation. The subjects of self-regulation and energy work are taboo in drug and scalpel medicine.

During the early 1980s, I suffered a headache on a flight from Jackson Hole, Wyoming, to Denver. By the time, I reached Denver to change my flight for Newark, the headache grew into a severe migraine attack. I decided to obtain relief with a Demerol injection. To my horror, I found out that rather than keep the drug in my briefcase as I always do, I had by mistake put it in my luggage checked for Newark. I knew no physician at the airport clinic, if any were immediately available, would give me a Demerol injection without doing a clinical evaluation and performing many laboratory tests. Furthermore, I would have to miss my flight to Newark. Terrified by the prospect of suffering a severe migraine headache all the way from Denver to Newark, I saw no way around it. I suffered severe pain and vomited and retched all through the insufferably long flight. At Newark airport I didn't care who saw me at the luggage area. As soon as I got my hands on the luggage, I pulled out the Demerol ampule and shot into me the full amount—usually half that amount suffices. An associate who had accompanied me to Jackson Hole drove me home.

Until I returned to clinical medicine in 1986, I did not face serious difficulties in managing my work since there were always other residents or pathology associates to take over when I became disabled. This changed when I began solo practice of immunology, environmental medicine and nutrition in 1986. Then a migraine headache attack forced me to cancel my office hours even when I knew some patients had traveled long distances to see me.

One early afternoon, I felt the heaviness in my head come on. I knew this would become a full-blown migraine attack and that my schedule was packed until midnight. It was a disconcerting thought. I wondered what it would mean for all the staff and patients if I had to cancel my hours. My discomfort grew into worry, then anxiety. It was then that the thought of trying autoregulation for brief periods but with high frequency crossed my mind. Frightened by the prospect of almost 12 hours of work with a migraine, I did pulses and limbic breathing frequently and earnestly.

The heaviness in my head didn't let up; instead, it turned into a headache. I vacillated about whether I should call the office staff and ask them to cancel my appointments or whether I should take the chance. In the past taking the chance meant keeping the early appointments and canceling the later ones as my migraine progressed. I remember many an occasion when I drove back home late at night, stopping a few times on the highway because I couldn't hold back the vomiting.

I persisted with autoregulation. Every 10 to 15 minutes, I did limbic breathing or tried doing pulses, a minute or two at a time. Such autoregulation seemed to have no impact on my headache at all. Still, I persisted. At about 5 p.m., I left the hospital and drove to the Institute, doing autoregulation all the way. As the migraine intensified, my anxiety grew. Within an hour or two, I realized the minute-reg made no difference and that the migraine would soon disable me. Close to despair, I decided to test my limits at both suffering from severe headaches and enduring autoreg. Somehow I managed to see my last patient and drive back home. It was close to midnight. My experiment with autoregulation done frequently but mostly for brief periods of time had obviously failed, creating new doubts about the very notion of autoregulation.

Once in my bedroom, I pulled out a Demerol vial and withdrew 2 ml of the drug into a syringe. At the last minute, something stopped me from shooting the narcotic into my vein. Instead, I lay down on my bed in the darkness and began limbic breathing for the nth time. The migraine slowly decreased in intensity and several minutes later it was completely gone. *This was the very first time in my memory that a full-blown migraine had cleared without a Demerol injection.*

On the third day after the migraine attack, I wondered why my migraine had cleared without the Demerol injection. Like a flash came the idea that it had to have been the autoregulation that I did for brief periods but with high frequency. I hadn't recognized this aspect of autoregulation by then.

The essential insight that experience gave me was this: The benefits of self-regulation may be delayed, but they are there. Autoregulation, done for a minute or two at a time, may not yield perceptible rewards at that time, but the cumulative energy responses and physiologic benefits that follow from them do add up.

MINUTE-REG AT WORK

"Minute-reg" is the term I use to describe a minute or two of autoregulation. The idea behind minute-reg is simple, and is to use some method of self-regulation for brief periods of time but with high frequency. It was through personal experiences like the one described above that I developed a deep sense of the great value of minute-reg in my autoregulation program.

Next, it seemed necessary to experiment further with minute-reg myself and define some aspects of its clinical usefulness before I could prescribe it to my patients.

Minute-reg gives the body tissues a respite from the unending demands of the cortical monkey. Even when it is as short as one to two minutes, a successful break like this interrupts the continual waves of biologic stress response that most of us face at work and at home every day.

After some time I became proficient at minute-reg. I was able to feel clear pulses in my fingertips almost instantaneously whenever I so desired.

ESCAPING INTO THE LIMBIC

In December 1986, I finished serving two terms as the elected president of Holy Name Hospital Medical Staff. The medical staff graciously decided to honor me for my service at a formal dinner scheduled for 7 p.m., I was expected to make some remarks after the dinner. In the past, I had known my predecessors to make prepared remarks in expressing their gratitude for the support they received during their terms of office as well as for the graciousness of the staff in honoring their work. I wondered about what I might prepare but couldn't come up with anything appropriate. I knew there were to be some other speakers and that many of them were going to roast me. So I decided to go along with whatever they might have to say and limit myself to responding to them in kind.

The day of the occasion was my day to examine all surgical specimens and perform frozen section biopsies for patients undergoing surgery. I planned to finish my work by 5 PM, then go home to shower and leave for the occasion. My morning work with surgical tissues was repeated interrupted by some problems in the laboratory. At about noon time I became aware of heaviness in my head that usually serves as an aura of my migraine headache attacks. The thought of having a migraine attack on the evening when I was to be the guest of honor horrified me. I fervently hoped that if I did minute-reg frequently all day long, perhaps I could abort the migraine attack. It turned out to be wishful thinking and the heaviness turned into dull headache within an hour. I thought about exchanging my day responsibilities with one of my associate pathologist, but decided against it. It realized it was a mistake when by 3 PM, my dull ache grew in intensity. Still, I persisted in my hope that I will finish my surgical work within an hour and have an hour to rest up.

I finished my laboratory work by 5 p.m. in the midst of a raging migraine attack accompanied with severe nausea. I was infuriated at myself for not having recognized the futility of my wishful thinking and for not having asked an associate to finish my work earlier during the afternoon when I might have had a chance of resting and abating my severe pain. What a silly mistake! What an embarrassment! I tried to control the surge of anger within me. I knew it would only make matters worse. Perhaps it was intense pain that clouded my judgment, I tried to reason with myself and mitigate my anger.

I became nauseated and my anxiety turned into panic as I

realized I had to somehow contact Mahmood Bangash, M.D., then chief of thoracic surgery who was moderating the occasion, and explain to him why I couldn't join them for the evening when they were to honor me. I realized he was in no position to call off the dinner. Dr. Bangash would simply have to announce that I had been disabled by a migraine attack. What a way to end my two terms of presidency of the medical staff!! Could I swing it with a Demerol injection? I wondered. No chance, the answer came readily. In the past, Demerol injections had totally disabled me and I had to be confined to the bed for several hours. I picked up the phone to call Dr. Bangash but put it back, afraid that my nausea might erupt into explosive vomiting during the call.

Desperate for some relief of pain and some way to save the evening, I locked my office, pulled out the telephone plug, laid down on the sofa, closed my eyes and started limbic breathing. The throbbing pain became more acute as I closed my eyes. Relaxation with slow breathing evidently was producing an effect opposite to what I had hoped. I thought about the day when I had succeeded in dissolving my migraine attack at my office without a Demerol injection. Why couldn't that day be today? I wailed. Some time later, I looked at the watch. It was about 5.30 p.m., and there was no sign of relief.

I have no memory of what happened during the next hour. What I do remember vividly is that I suddenly sat up on the sofa, my hands trembling, my face flushed, my forehead sweating. Frightened and disoriented, I shook my head as I recovered from some very distressing sensations I had experienced moments earlier. I had felt as if I was being dismembered. In that dazed state, I had not seen any blood nor any gaping wounds. But the clear and extremely frightening sense was of my limbs separating and floating away from my torso. With my eyes I had seen myself fragmented.

Moments later, I felt relief as I assured myself that that frightening experience was nothing more than a nightmare. Several moments later, suddenly I realized that my headache had completely disappeared. I touched my forehead in confusion, then moved my fingers through my hair—not certain whether the relief was real or imagined. Slowly I realized that my migraine attack indeed had abated and that I could stand up and move about the room to gather some strength. I stood up, stretched and slowly took some steps to make certain that I don't quickly become dizzy as I had done on numerous previous occasions after a migraine attack. I felt neither weak nor dizzy. I looked at the watch. It was a few minutes to 7 p.m. Encouraged by my ability to walk around without any symptoms, I prepared to leave my office. With not enough time to go home to shower, I washed my face in the office sink, picked up my briefcase and walked out to be at the dinner.

There were the expected speeches by some friends. They roasted me for my vagrant ideas about the impact of environment on human biology and poked fun at me (a pathologist) trying to play a doctor in the evening. In the end, I was expected to thank them for their kindness and grace and find a way to make them laugh. I did that. (No, I didn't say anything about N^2D^2 medicine. There is a time and a place for everything, I told myself.) If anyone noticed anything different in me that evening, they didn't tell me.

The following day, I decided to call whatever I had experienced a *limbic break*. In autoregulation lingo, it meant a sudden escape from the relentless terror of the thinking mind—an entry into the limbic openness where the arteries have no reason to stay tightened. The muscles have no cause to be in spasm. The body tension simply melts away. The cortical monkey is banished. There is no reason for a headache anymore.

During the period of disorientation when I had experienced the feeling of dismemberment, I had no sense that such an experience might be called an out-of-body experience by others. Or, more precisely, it may be considered a form of what has been called *kundalini* in India for millennia. What name to give it didn't seem important. Now, almost nine years after it happened, I clearly see that what I experienced that day was what millions of others have experienced in their lives. These are moments of sudden and merciful withdrawal from the unremitting agony of the thinking mind—times when the cortical monkey is stopped dead in his tracks and can no more mercilessly beat up on injured tissues. Whatever anyone chooses to call it is okay with me.

Could I simply have dozed off? Could my migraine attack have simply subsided in sleep? I know that is not true. I have suffered too many times when I went to bed with a headache and woke up with a headache eight hours later to believe that simply dozing off broke the hold of this migraine.

A TIME FOR TRUTH

Several months after the episode of limbic break I describe above, one late evening I was to fly to Denver to speak at the annual meeting of the American Academy of Environmental Medicine. I planned to finish my laboratory work at the hospital, then see several patients at the Institute before leaving for Newark airport. At about 5 p.m., before I left the hospital, I began to feel my migraine aura of head heaviness. By then, I had dissolved my migraine on several occasions and had become somewhat arrogant about my capacity for doing so. I thought I would do minute-reg in between seeing patients, do frequent limbic breathing, and speed up my schedule so as to have some time to dissolve my migraine attack before leaving for the airport. Talat was flying with me and that gave me some comfort. Under the worst circumstances, I could ask her to drive and I would do autoregulation myself during the ride to the airport.

As is often the case with my schedule, some patients required more time than I thought they would. Rather than speeding up my schedule, I fell behind. The intensity of my headache grew and I developed nausea. Talat kept sending me messages that we were getting very tight on time and that seemed to feed my headache further. By the time we left the office, I had a full-blown migraine attack. I asked Talat to drive. Even before we could get onto the Garden State Parkway, I felt a strong vomiting reflex and asked her to pull over. She did so and offered me tissue paper to clean up after I threw up on the roadside. She had done so on more occasions than she cared to count.

During the ride, I breathed limbically and thought about how many migraine attacks I had dissolved with autoregulation previously. The intensity of the pain, however, didn't let up. Still, I felt secure that eventually I would be able to break this attack just as I had done on many occasions. I continued to experience nausea and retching as we parked the car at the airport. Somehow I managed to walk through the terminal without stopping to vomit again. At the counter line, I struggled to suppress my retching. Once in a window seat in the plane, I felt secure in the knowledge that I could discreetly relieve persistent nausea by vomiting if I had to without making an ugly scene for many to watch.

Minutes passed. The plane taxied to the runway, then flew up through thin clouds illuminated by a lowering sun. My migraine raged on. I don't remember now how long it took before the intensity of suffering began to break down my resolve to dissolve the pain with autoregulation. It had been more than two hours since I threw up by the roadside in Bloomfield. I had tried limbic breathing, tissue sensing, shrinking circles (a method I find useful for controlling headache), and many other techniques to control my pain. Nothing had worked. I even tried directed pulses—something I caution my patients not to do during a headache. The pulses only made my pain more acute. Exhausted and dejected, I considered administering myself a Demerol injection, then backed off. Many more minutes of agony passed. There was no relief in sight. I asked Talat to take out Demerol from my briefcase. (For years, I hadn't dared to travel without Demerol in my briefcase.) She pulled out the drug into a syringe, taking precaution not to let any passengers see it. I took the syringe from her and felt a tremendous relief simply looking at it.

A thought hit me as I prepared to plunge the needle into my flesh: Do it, but if you do, you will never teach autoregulation to anyone. I stopped and lowered the hand carrying the syringe. The thought continued: If you take the shot now, you will throw out the autoregulation equipment. Get out of this work. You have *no* right to teach this to patients with multiple sclerosis, lupus, crippling rheumatoid arthritis and cancer, if you cannot dissolve a mere migraine with it yourself. If this is deception, it must end. And it must end *today*. Go on. Get your Demerol fix. But don't live with this lie again.

I looked out the window. Everything looked hazy through the pain in my eyes. I gave the syringe back to Talat, covered my face with my hands, and wondered whether crying would help.

My next memory of that day is of the greatest "high" I have ever experienced in autoregulation. It was the most intense energy experience ever in my life. The clouds up near the sinking sun were crimson. I had never seen that crimson before nor have I since that time. The pale blue sky was luminous. I had never seen luminous sky like that earlier, nor since. The space where heaven lifts up the earth was wide open, wider than I ever saw. The *presence* there was larger than I had ever seen.

HEADACHES AND PULSES

Aside from chronic headaches caused by musculoskeletal problems of the neck and shoulder, all chronic headaches—in my view—are caused by sensitivity to molds, foods and chemicals. Stress exaggerates headaches only in those who are vulnerable to the sensitivities in the first place. Brain tumors and metabolic disorders do not cause the common types of chronic headaches and migraines.

Optimal management of allergies and chemical sensitivities can relieve headaches 80 to 90 percent of the time. For complete control of chronic headaches, in my extensive clinical experience (as well as that of an ex-migraine patient), some effective methods of self-regulation are essential.

TWO IMPORTANT POINTS

I want to make two important points here. First, headaches almost always become worse when the sufferer begins to do any type of self-regulation. Autoregulation is no exception. Countless patients have corroborated my own earlier experience with this phenomenon that I describe above. It is easy to understand. Closing eyes to do autoregulation cancels out many extraneous factors that often detract from pain perception. So temporarily the pain gains in intensity. There is only one right thing to do in such a state: hang on and persist with autoregulation.

Second, pulses may not be a good method for self-regulation in the control of headaches. The reason for this is simple. Headaches almost always are associated with spasms and, in later stages, with persistent dilatation of arteries. Such changes may indeed be worsened by the method of pulses. I do not consider it advisable to direct pulses to eyes or any part of the head for headache control. The best autoregulation methods for the control of headache are limbic breathing and limbic energy work.

JEFFERSON'S HEADACHE

When I first came to this country, Thomas Jefferson fascinated me more than any other president. Talat and I visited Monticello on several occasions before our children were born, then with our children when they were old enough to learn the history of the United States. I read his writings and wondered about how the tall young man with a freckled face and red hair might have walked around in the woods by Monticello, and later as an old man with gray hair after he retired from public office.

Jefferson suffered migraine headaches. Sometimes his pain was so intense that he stayed holed up in a dark room at Monticello for days. Thanks to Demerol and Vistaril injections, I never suffered from my migraine attacks that long. But I remember thinking about Jefferson's misery when I stayed holed up in a dark room trying to obtain some relief from my headache before I finally succumbed and used the Demerol injection to put myself out. How did Jefferson cope with his headache for days? I couldn't imagine. How often did he suffer migraine attacks when he went to the Virginia House of Burgesses? And when he wrote the Declaration of Independence? And when he was in Paris seeking French support? And, finally, when he was the president of the United States? Perhaps his years in Paris were symptom-free. Perhaps he didn't have any migraine attacks at all during his years in the White House. I have been told that migraine attack subside with advancing age.

Sometimes when I suffered my migraine attacks I thought about Jefferson's pain and felt a strange kinship with him. I remember the many times I joked about how I never wanted anyone to cure my migraine headaches. That seemed to be the only true link I had with Thomas Jefferson.

Years later, with autoregulation I learned to escape into a limbic state where there are no migraine attacks and no need for Demerol or Vistaril shots. Repeated personal experiences convinced me that autoregulation was not a placebo the effects of which would be expected to wear off with time. Then I proceeded to teach hundreds of migraine headache sufferers methods of escaping the tyranny of the thinking mind—and that of migraine headaches.

Sometimes I wondered if I could have taught Thomas Jefferson to dissolve his migraine headaches the way I did mine. I would have to run some tests for mold allergy and food sensitivities. (I'm certain he had some, because to date I have never seen a patient who suffers migraine headaches who doesn't have provable mold and food sensitivities.) I would have had no difficulty effectively managing Jefferson's allergies. From reading about him, I feel he probably also suffered from sugar dysregulation—sugar-insulin-adrenaline-neurotransmitter roller coasters are seen in almost all cases of migraine. Of course, I have no way of knowing, but I think I would have succeeded. A man of his towering intellect, I know, would have had no difficulty understanding the true nature of self-regulation and learning how to turn his unrelenting mind off with limbic breathing and mitigate his suffering.

If only Jefferson could return, I could prove myself right!

ACUTE BACKACHE AT THE MET

During my mid-thirties, I often suffered from chronic neck pain and backache—a professional hazard for pathologists who are not careful about their posture at the microscope. When I began my work with preventive medicine, I did not want to preach anything that I didn't practice myself. During my writing of *The*

Ghoraa and Limbic Exercise, I experimented with many different exercises for chronic neck pain and backache. I chose some that I found effective on a regular basis. During that period I learned some stretching exercises that completely relieved my neck and back pain.

Then one day my backache returned. First it was intermittent, not severe enough to keep me from maintaining my regular schedule. Within days it grew in intensity. Then Talat and I went to the Virgin Islands for a vacation. My backache worsened with the travel. I realized I needed to have some X-rays and a MRI scan of the back done to make sure that it was all due to muscle spasms and pulled ligaments rather than some structural damage to the disc, or worse, a growth in the spinal cord. On our return, I delayed the MRI scan for a few days. The following weekend, while rambling along at the Metropolitan Museum of Art, I was suddenly struck by a sharp pain. I froze on the spot, as even the slightest movement caused excruciating pain in my back. I felt angry at myself for having neglected the back problem and wondered how I would manage to get to the hospital for an MRI scan without calling an ambulance. Nearly in panic, I thought of relieving the acute muscle spasm in my back with autoregulation.

I do not recall how long it took, but I was able to walk out of the museum and walk back to our apartment in the city. Once again as my back pain subsided I deferred the MRI scan. I wanted to test if gentle limbic exercise and autoregulation could resolve my back problem. That episode occurred more than three years ago. I neither underwent the scans nor needed to see a physician. Occasionally, I feel some muscle spasm and pain in my lower back. Some stretching exercises and limbic breathing are all I need for relief.

CHEST PAIN ON BROADWAY

On another occasion, Talat and I went for a walk on Broadway in New York City. I woke up fresh and well rested that morning. I did my usual morning limbic stretching and limbic run. I didn't feel any muscular stress in the chest muscles or anywhere else. On Broadway, out of the blue, came a sense of discomfort in the chest. We continued to walk and I decided not to say anything about it to Talat. Several minutes later, I realized that the discomfort was turning out actual pain and it seemed to be localizing in the left chest. I stopped for a few moments on the pretense of looking at books in the display windows of Barnes and Noble on 81st Street. The pain seemed to ease off. We resumed our walk and pain returned. This happened a few times before I felt a sense of concern.

Several minutes later, the sense of concern turned into one of alarm. Even though I do not have any defined risk factors for heart disease, I had done too many autopsies on patients who died of a heart attack and who had no definable risk factors. Their heart attacks were mistaken for indigestion or muscle spasm. I suggested to Talat that we should sit on one of the benches on the Broadway divider strip and watch people. My real purpose was to not ignore the chest pain. I decided to either dissolve it with autoregulation completely or tell Talat about it and return to Teaneck for a cardiogram and some other tests. If it were a muscle spasm in the chest wall or an esophageal reflux, I reasoned, I should be able to terminate that with autoregulation. I further thought that since most heart attacks are caused by the spasm of the coronary heart arteries in the beginning, autoregulation would benefit that as well.

I do not recall how long it took me to completely dissolve my chest pain. It may have been 15 minutes or more. The pain never returned. I didn't require any cardiac evaluation, neither then nor since.

IRREVERSIBLE PULPITIS AT DELPHI

Once while traveling in the countryside of Greece, I developed an acute toothache. Rather than return to Athens for dental care, I decided to wing it. The next day, when we reached Delphi, my pain grew in intensity and made it impossible for me even to eat soup. I tapped a tooth on my right side with a spoon—just as my endodontist had done on three previous occasions to diagnose a root canal problem—and convulsed with sharp pain. "Irreversible pulpitis," I recalled his words when I had experienced exactly the same type of pain in his office. I felt a panic as I realized that we were to travel for three more days before our scheduled arrival in Athens where I could reach an endodontist. I thought about discussing the need for terminating our trip with Talat, then changed my mind. Let's see what the next day brings, I told myself. I began doing autoregulation and stayed with it almost without interruption except to briefly answer Talat's questions. Subsisting on fluids, I managed the pain until we returned to Athens. Once secure in the knowledge that I could see an endodontist at short notice, I decided to test an idea: Can irreversible pulpitis be reversed?

It has been more than four years since that time of

irreversible pulpitis. I still have my tooth and I haven't had a root canal. (I am much more careful with my dental care and am very grateful for the care I have received from my excellent endodontist and periodontist since that time.) Several months ago, my periodontist suggested that I have another tooth removed that she thought was beyond salvation. I asked her if she would support me in my efforts to conserve the tooth. She smiled and consented. (I still have that tooth.)

SPONTANEITY OF PULSES

Serendipity opened my eyes to the enormous value of pulses for dissolving anger.

One day at the hospital, a technician brought me an unlabeled frozen section surgical biopsy slide. A frozen section study of the fresh biopsy specimen is undertaken so that the pathologist can render a definitive diagnosis to the operating surgeon while the patient is still in the operating room. It allows the surgeon to make a judgment about the type of operation to be performed and the amount of healthy tissue which must be sacrificed to assure complete removal of the cancer. Not uncommonly, two or more surgeons send their biopsies to the laboratory at the same time. Thus it is critically important that the biopsy specimens be processed separately and the slides prepared with the biopsy materials be labeled accurately and immediately. Errors in mislabeling slides—or not labeling them immediately—can have disastrous consequences for the patient. Safety in this area is always a top priority for surgical pathologists.

This had been a very busy morning. There had been several frozen section studies, and I had been distracted by staff in other areas of the laboratory. (We pathologists repeatedly remind ourselves of the potential for serious error when we are distracted during microscopic work.) I recognized the unlabeled frozen section slide and suddenly became furious. I asked a staff member to immediately call that technician and ask him to come to my office. The technician got wind of my anger and disappeared for lunch. I felt the anger in full swing now. This is when it happened.

Suddenly, and certainly without a conscious effort on my part, the pulses arrived at my fingertips. My hands felt flushed. Suddenly my neck muscles were limp, my legs and feet light. I sensed something move through my entire body with the speed of lightening, yet gently. The tension in my muscles melted away, as if all the tightness wrung into my tissues by the surge of anger was simply swept clean—as if, caught in cortical clutches as I was, an ethereal limbic wave set me free. All of a sudden, I found myself in a comforting limbic openness—and smiling at myself. I was not angry anymore. I thought about the technician at lunch and wondered how his digestive juices might be working since he knew he couldn't stay away from the laboratory—and me—forever.

How did the pulses know I needed them? Where did they come from? Certainly the subject of pulses couldn't have been further from my mind in those moments of fury. Which part of my *being* sensed my predicament? How did that part order the pulses around? Was it my thinking mind or some other dimension of the mind that eludes the thinking mind? Or was it not the doing of mind at all? Did the muscles in the arterial walls let go by themselves? Did the cells lining the inside of the blood vessels suddenly feel some sympathy for me? Did they abruptly decide to splurge their nitric oxide and endothelin stores—the simple molecules that endothelial cells in the vessel walls produce to free the tightened vessels from the unrelenting dictates of the thinking mind? I looked out the window and laughed out loud as I acknowledged the volley of questions from my conscious mind. Of course, the conscious mind had no answer for any of them.

Months later, I became curious to learn if any of my patients who did autoregulation regularly ever experienced such limbic breaks. Many of them did, but each did so in his own way. *The limbic has its own sense of beings.*

THE RETURN OF MIGRAINE

From 1991 to 1996, I didn't need to administer Demerol and Vistaril injections to myself to control pain. I had become quite proficient in dissolving my migraine attacks with autoregulation. I found limbic breathing especially useful for them. Then I began to wonder if my long period of relief had more to do with my advancing age rather than with my success with autoregulation. One mellows with age and so may be expected to be less susceptible to the Fourth-of-July chemistry that feeds the fires of migraine attacks. In the fall of 1996 I got my answer. I suffered such a severe migraine attack that despite all attempts to control it, I had to inject myself with the drugs to control pain. While giving myself the injections I experienced the additional frustration of breaking the long spell of my injection-free period, but my pain was simply unbearable. There was also the disturbing sense that I wouldn't be able to relate to my patients anymore my own case history and victory over migraine headache.

The rising sun the next morning during my limbic run gave me a newer perspective. Wasn't the fact that I still suffered an unbearable migraine headache attack after all those years of relief the proof that the control of pain had more to do with my success with limbic breathing than with my advancing age. I found the thought comforting. I felt reassured that after all I could attribute my success to autoregulation, and to my advancing age. My thoughts returned to Jefferson. Perhaps he did suffer migraine attacks while in the White House.

****

In closing this chapter, I wish to emphasize that facility with self-regulation and energy work is a gift from God. It comes easily to some and with considerable difficulty to others. Each of us must recognize this. Each of us has some strengths and some weaknesses. What matters in work with self-regulation and spirituality is this: Everyone eventually succeeds, at his own time, at his own pace. We must accept this. Being goal-oriented, competitive, or combative doesn't help.

"Winning isn't everything, it's the *only* thing," the American guru of competitiveness, Vince Lombardi, exhorted his disciples. We must recognize that Lombardi philosophy of winning is utterly irrelevant to matters of healing and spirituality.

Thinking is an intellectual function; healing isn't. In autoregulation, I do not ask my patients to think positively. Rather, I strive to teach them how not to think. Thinking about how not to think is a classical catch 22; the harder we try not to think, the deeper we slide into thinking.

The Cortical Monkey and Healing

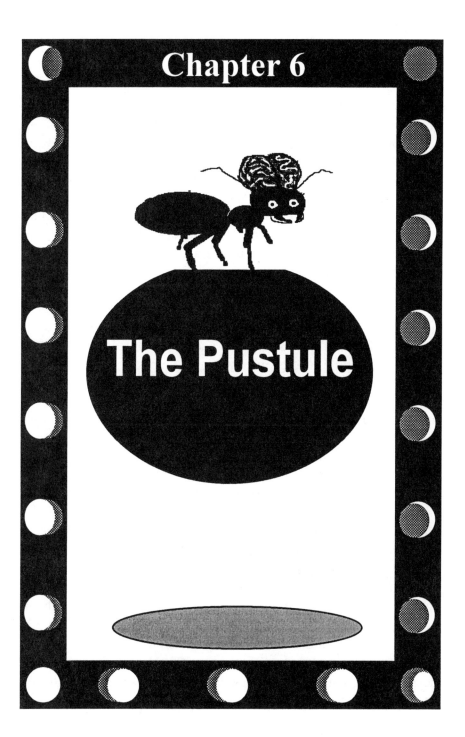

Chapter 6

The Pustule

In January 1995, I nicked the skin of my upper lip while shaving. The tiny cut stopped bleeding after a few minutes. But the next morning, my blade shaved off the tiny scab at the site of the nick and caused more bleeding. I carefully avoided injuring the scab the following morning, but to my annoyance, abraded it yet again. The nick bled even more than it had earlier. After my shower, I gently wiped the tiny blood clot at the site of the nick and noticed red swelling underneath. I decided to use a pair of fine scissors to clip the hair around this area rather than use a razor blade until it healed completely.

For a few mornings, I carefully shaved around the lesion and clipped the hair around it with scissors. The papule began to shrink and its redness subsided. Then one morning I nicked it again. The papule bled profusely. Some words of frustration rose to my lips. I stopped the bleeding by applying direct pressure over the cut for several minutes. During mid-morning I noticed a blood stain on my shirt and wondered how the blood reached from my face to my shirt. That evening the papule had grown further in size. A granuloma! I muttered to myself with annoyance. A granuloma is a pimple composed of rich vascular repair tissue that bleeds readily with minor trauma.

In the following weeks, I diligently avoided nicking the granuloma on most days but failed to do so on others. The papule seemed to shrink on some days, then grow on others. One day a droplet of gray-white pus appeared just below the surface of the papule and the skin at its periphery had turned deep red and edematous. So now the stupid thing has turned into a granuloma pyogenicum! I murmured with consternation. In pathologic terminology, a granuloma that doesn't heal, bleeds easily, and accumulates purulent fluid within it is called a pyogenic granuloma. I realized that by sheer carelessness I had turned a simple, quick-healing shaving nick into a pyogenic granuloma. It annoyed me further to recognize that the lesion would leave behind an ugly scar when it healed.

How long will I have to wear this silly thing on my face to the hospital? And how long will I exhibit it to my patients at the Institute? I wondered. What irked me most about the granuloma was that I had to display it on my face during my weekly autoregulation workshops. I taught the principles and practice of autoregulation to my patients in those workshops. The first method I usually teach is directed pulses, and the first clinical application I often talk about is the possibility of healing common injuries and inflammatory lumps with directed pulses. Wouldn't the students see an ugly, purulent pimple on my face day after day and wonder why the miracle of directed pulses didn't work for the teacher himself? That question was disconcerting. I decided to get serious about the pyogenic granuloma and rid myself of it with autoregulation.

While driving to the hospital that morning and to the Institute that afternoon, I sent directed pulses to my papule. The next morning I looked into the mirror and studied the lesion. There was no pus, and the lesion seemed to have shrunken a bit—at least that's what I saw or imagined. Wow! That's something. I was like the cat who swallowed a canary. This stuff really works! A few more sessions with directed pulses and I'll wipe the whole silly thing off my face. And when that happens, I told myself, I'll have another autoregulation story to add to my miracle book.

THE PRURIENT PUSTULE

The next morning I studied the granuloma, as a cat might a chicken once she has found a way into the chicken coop. One more day, perhaps two, and that's all you're worth, I told the granuloma confidently. Again I performed autoreg, sending pulses to the granuloma during my morning ride to the hospital and as I rode to the Institute in the afternoon. The morning after, I jumped out of bed and rushed to the mirror to see the miserable state of my hapless victim—the granuloma. What I saw there disgusted me: The granuloma looked uglier, angrier and pussier. It had turned into a pustule. What's that! I nearly yelled at the mirror. Within moments I recovered and stared at the ugly thing. Then it began to itch. Ever so gently I rubbed it, but it bled and itched even more. I put a drop of cold water on it. It itched more. "You, prurient little pustule!" I yelled at the lesion. "I see now you're not going to go away like that! But I'll fix you," I told the pustule defiantly. "Autoregulation during driving time may not be enough for you. But you watch!"

I started sending pulses to my upper lip during my morning limbic runs—I suppose I didn't want to dignify the pustule by addressing it directly. Limbic running is a type of nongoal-oriented, noncompetitive, meditative run that is a part of my morning meditation. I describe limbic running fully in the companion volume *The Ghoraa and Limbic Exercise*.

MY PRIVATE WAR BEGINS

Days passed, but the pustule didn't clear up. On some days, I thought—or perhaps imagined—I was winning, but then the pustule would grow back. One day pus in the pustule was too visible to be tolerated, so with a sterile needle I let it out. That afternoon the pustule went down. But that was not what I wanted. I was once a surgeon and wasn't about to be impressed by a pustule shrinking after the pus within it was let out. What I was determined to do was to clear the ugly mess *energetically* and *limbically*. The pustule seemed to taunt me: "That's not what autoregulation is all about. Any dummy can let out the pocket of pus in me and I will shrink." The pustule mocked: "You boast that your autoregulation is about energy healing. Why don't you try some other clever scheme?" My conversation with the pustule was becoming more annoying by the moment. Of course, the pustule was right. The mechanical removal of pus wasn't what I desired.

In the days that followed, I continued directing pulses to my upper lip whenever I could. Sometime later, the pus cleared and the pustule shrank. Then one day I nicked the granuloma again and restarted the whole process. The pus reappeared promptly—or perhaps the razor nick might have brought it out from within some deep recess. Disillusioned, I thought about some other strategy of self-regulation that might prove effective in my private war against the pustule.

Until then I had been smug in my belief that, given sufficient time, I could melt away little lumps and bumps at will with directed pulses. The defiant pustule seemed to be changing all that. The memory of dissolving a chalazion in my eyelid with directed pulses was still fresh in my mind. From a pathologic standpoint, dissolving a chalazion with directed pulses seemed utterly logical and scientific—not at all the stuff that miracles are made of. Furthermore, dissolution of an indolent chalazion was a far tougher project than clearing a pyogenic granuloma.

Until my pustule shattered my conviction about the efficacy of directed pulses, my only problem had been how to teach effectively the theory of such pulses to my patients and how to guide them through practical sessions. Now it was different. The prurient pustule was threatening my conviction. It loomed as proof of my frivolous thinking—proof I *had* to wear on my face at all times and *had* to see whenever I looked into the mirror.

Vexed at the pustule, I began to consider the possibility of a surgical excision of the pustule, but each time I firmly ruled out that option. I told myself that I had not given autoregulation a real chance. *How often do you ask your patients to keep trying when autoregulation doesn't work initially?* I reminded myself each time the thought of surgery crossed my mind.

As the pustule persisted, some of the staff at the hospital sympathetically inquired about the lesion. Some offered me their diagnostic options—including the possibility of skin cancer—and wondered when I was going to have it burned off by cautery. I good-naturedly fielded their questions and reassured them that I was sure it was a benign granuloma that had developed at the site of repeated shaving nicks. And further, I assured them that I wasn't worried about it.

One day in the laboratory hallway, my associate

pathologists, Evelynne Braun, M.D., and Verna Atkins, M.D., carefully examined my pyogenic granuloma. They, of course, knew of my interest in energy work and about my failed attempts to clear the granuloma with directed pulses. In unison and with clinical authority, they pronounced that the granuloma wouldn't heal with directed pulses or with any other form of chicanery. Some histology technicians joined them, and all of them told me that the lesion on my face was ugly and unbecoming of a laboratory director. It was all in good humor, and I acknowledged the earnest advice of my staff like a good chief pathologist.

Then Ronald Remy, M.D., Director of Surgery at the hospital, walked into the laboratory corridor in the company of his associate, John Poole, M.D. Dr. Atkins, who had been the more vociferous of the group, asked the two surgeons to examine my face and render their diagnoses—hoping it might add weight to her recommendation of surgical excision. One of the surgeons thought it was a wart and the other deemed it a shaving cut turned into a granuloma. I tried to be a good sport and listened to their comments attentively. Next, Dr. Remy graciously invited me to walk over to the operating suites with him right then so that he could burn the granuloma off with a cautery, using a few drops of local anesthetic. I thanked him for his kind interest in my predicament but declined his offer for surgical removal of the pustule.

Some weeks later, in early March, Talat and I visited Kenya at the invitation of our daughter, Sarah, who was there for her fellowship after receiving her master's degree from the Harvard School of Public Health. The long plane trip offered me an opportunity to direct pulses to the pustule for extended periods of time. Once on the safari in Kenya, I knew I would have all the necessary time to perform autoreg. I was confident I would succeed and be able to dissolve the pustule with directed energy work. To make certain that I wouldn't nick the wound during shaving, I decided to grow a moustache and beard. My strategy seemed surefire.

The manuscript of this book—except for this chapter entitled The Pustule—was nearly complete. I packed it in my luggage in the hope that there would be enough time for me to make some minor, final changes before submitting it for publication on my return. The flights from New York to Jedda and Nairobi, as expected, gave me much time to direct pulses to the pustule as well as to do work on the manuscript. We spent fabulous days on our safari in Masai Mara Game Reserve and other parks in northern Kenya where the wildlife was enchanting. Of course, there was enough time to do as much autoregulation for my pustule as I wanted.

On my return to the U.S., I shaved and found, to my chagrin, that the granuloma had not healed. Rather, its surface was encrusted harder during the days it was protected by the growth of hair around it. It was an annoying and humiliating sight. All that work with directed pulses had been in vain. I felt cheated, and for some brief moments my confidence in the efficacy of self-regulation in clinical medicine was shattered.

Why didn't the pulses work? That question haunted me. I realized that a pyogenic granuloma is a highly vascular lesion and began to wonder if it had been wise to send yet more blood with directed pulses to an area already drenched with blood. I began to think of some other approach. Would some sort of directed imagery like a laser beam work? I wondered. I tried directed imagery a few times, then realized it was the work of the trickster cortical monkey and abandoned the effort.

Weeks passed. As had happened before the Kenya trip, sometimes the granuloma shrank, then grew again. In spite of my best efforts not to lacerate the pustule during shaving, I nicked it every now and then. Each time it seemed to bleed more profusely than before. Some more months passed and I tried to reconcile with the granuloma. It will heal when it chooses to do so, I told myself. The thoughts of surgical removal, burning the lesion with cautery, or clearing it with some salve returned several times. Each time I decided not to act, and the granuloma prevailed.

Each morning the granuloma was a reminder of my failure. The staff at the hospital and the Institute often made passing remarks about it. Each Monday when I conducted an autoregulation workshop, I was conscious of the ugly, red purulent pustule on my face. I knew my patients noticed it but were too polite to refer to it as I taught them directed pulses to facilitate healing.

In the fall of that year, almost ten months after the pustule developed, I began work on a series of 20 Life Span Videos. Some videos were designed to cover the broad subjects of nutrition, environment, stress, exercise and healing, while others were devoted to specific disorders such as asthma, cancer, fatigue, heart disease, and hyperactivity, among others. I knew there were to be many close-up shots of my face during that series of videos and that my pyogenic granuloma would be clearly visible to the viewers. I also recognized that, once completed, those videos would be copied many times for distribution. Furthermore, the time and effort required to complete the project would render a second recording unlikely if the appearance of the granuloma on close-up shots of my face was repulsive. Not only were those thoughts disconcerting for the possibility of duplicating that work, they were unpleasant reminders of my vanity. I seriously considered having the granuloma removed by a surgeon-friend, but as in the case of all previous such attempts, I was unable to act on that. Finally, I proceeded with the video project and completed the filming over the following five Saturdays. The granuloma showed clearly on my face, but no one at the Institute seemed to be concerned about it. I decided to ignore the granuloma.

But the granuloma refused to be ignored. It teased, provoked, and mocked me every time I looked into a mirror. As much as I wanted to withdraw myself from this unsolicited war, the pustule never let me. Sometimes I reminded myself of horrible malignant lesions I had seen on my patients' faces. At other times I thought about the terrible facial mutilations left by cancer surgery. What is this stupid granuloma compared to all that I have seen in others? I would console myself.

In January 1996, a year after I first recognized the lesion as a pyogenic granuloma, I made the final decision never to consider surgical removal or treatment with salves. I resigned myself to a life shared with my facial granuloma.

The problem for me was never the issue of discomfort or the mechanical aspects of surgery. I am a fully trained general surgeon. In 1966, fully 30 years earlier, I had passed the examination for the diploma of Fellow of the Royal College of Surgeons of England. During my years of practice in the art of surgery, I performed many operations and knew that excision of my granuloma would be completely safe. (Whenever I trivialize minor surgical operations by making comments such as the one above, I am reminded of a surgical axiom: There is no minor surgery, only minor surgeons.)

In September 1996, nearly 20 months after the appearance

of my blessed pyogenic granuloma, a young woman consulted me for disabling chronic fatigue and associated immune disorders. During the initial interview, she said, "Dr. Ali, I've tried many approaches with many doctors before. Nothing has helped me. I came to see you because I have read one of your books, and I know you do energy work. I hope you can help me *heal*. I was once very good at energy healing. Please believe me when I tell you that I once cleared a ganglion cyst on my wrist with energy work within one day." Before I knew it, I felt my right index and middle fingers cover my granuloma. Self-consciously and slowly I removed my hand from my face and carried on with the pretense of listening to her with rapt attention. Inside, I felt like a fake. How can I help you heal your entire badly damaged body defense system with energy when I can't wipe this simple, silly, ugly pustule from my face with energy work? I wanted to say that, but didn't. I let her continue until she moved on to other subjects. Then a very strange sense overwhelmed me. I knew the time had come for my pyogenic granuloma to clear up.

On our way back from the office, I told Talat that I knew the time for the pustule's dissolution had arrived. She gave me a confused glance. I had kept her fully informed about the details of my humiliating war with the pustule since I first recognized it as a granuloma 20 months earlier. She knew why I had stopped shaving during our Kenya trip 15 months earlier. She also knew that I had postponed applying the finishing touches to the manuscript of this volume *(Healing, Miracles and the Bite of the Gray Dog)* on my return from Kenya. I told her I couldn't complete the book without writing something about my privately lost war with my pustule.

How can I let the chapter entitled The Miracle of Directed Pulses get published while my pustule jeers at me every time I look into a mirror? I asked myself a thousand times during those months. Indeed, so great was my frustration with the pustule that I abandoned work on the manuscript that included chapters on directed pulses and instead wrote and published *What Do Lions Know About Stress?* during the year after our return from Kenya. That volume was inspired by a lion who limped many yards behind his harem of five sleek and sublime lionesses whom we were fortunate to have tracked for a few miles.

On that late evening driving home, I was confidently telling Talat that the time for my pustule to clear up had arrived. She had looked at me in silence. Some moments passed, and then her confused look turned into an amused smile. "When did that happen?" she asked. I had told her about my visit with the young woman who dissolved a ganglion cyst on her wrist with energy work, and then about the strange sense that I had about the imminent healing of the pustule. "We'll see," she said after I finished. The next day she left town to visit with her family.

The second night after my conversation with Talat, I woke up with a sharp stinging sensation in my face. I touched my face and found it was wet. I moved my hand around and realized the liquid reached down to my neck. I bolted up in my bed, confused. It took me a few moments to realize that the fluid that made my face and neck wet might be blood. I touched my pillow. A part of it was also wet. I rushed to the bathroom, turned the lights on, and found my face and neck covered with blood. Hurriedly I washed my face and neck. My eyes focused on my upper lip. The pustule was gone. There was a raw, oozing area at the bed of the pustule. I dried the raw area with a clean tissue, wondered what that had been all about, and returned to bed.

When Talat returned three days later, there was no sign of

anything ever having been there on my upper lip.

So today, January 5, 1997, I finish this chapter. Since September 1996, when my pustule bid me farewell, there has not been a single morning when I've shaved without remembering the pustule—without a sense of relief at not worrying about lacerating it or wasting time to cautiously shave around it, then pull out a pair of scissors to clip the hair around it. Shaving my upper lip is a breeze now. And something else is there. Each morning brings me a treasured gift of reflection and appreciation. Why did the pustule take 20 months to clear? Why didn't it heal earlier? And when finally it healed, why did it?

As I write this, my thoughts drift to Homer's Iliad. His gods were ambivalent about his Greek warriors who waged war against Troy for ten long years. The gods certainly vacillated much during the decade of war, supporting the Greek here and their enemies there. Even the Greek supergod, Zeus, remained indecisive and kept sending mixed signals to the Spartan and Athenian warriors. The Greek suffered heavy casualties at the hands of Troy, and lost most of their heros. Why couldn't Zeus make up his mind earlier? He could have ended the strife, and helped the Greek a little. And all that happened when the Greek were helping Menelaus, Zeus's own son-in-law, in his struggle to save his honor and free Helen—his wife, and daughter of Zeus and Lida—from Paris of Troy who had abducted her. Fierce Zeus was known to strike and dissipate mere mortals with his lightening rod for trivial offenses. Why did he let Paris dishonor his own daughter and get away with it for so long? And when he finally did come to Menelaus's rescue and burned down Troy, why did he? He had been awfully slow to come up with his plan to subvert the Tory by packing the best of the Greek warriors in the belly of his Trojan horse. What took him so long? Why such hurtful indecisiveness? That Homer, the poor rascal! His gods confounded him much.

Healing is a spontaneous process. My thoughts return to the pustule. What happened to the spontaneity of healing during those 20 months when my pustule refused stubbornly to heal? Years earlier, my chalazion healed rapidly with directed pulses. Why didn't the pustule dissolve with such pulses? What kept me from asking a surgeon-friend to burn off my pustule during all those months? What kept me from clearing that pustule with a salve? And when the pustule did leave me, why did it? What clues did it finally heed? *Who directed it?* The questions remain unanswered. At least I have that in common with Homer.

But my mornings are free of all questions. Each morning brings me a unique gift: one of remembrance of the pustule and of gratitude for my linkage with the larger *presence* that permeates and surrounds me at every moment. It is a reminder to me that the *presence* is not bound to my notions of healers and healing, and is not subordinate to my schedule. I shall *never* know the answer to the simple questions about why the pustule didn't heal for so long and why it did when it did.

I now see that my pustule was a gift to me, to be treasured and remembered. Would my pustule be as precious a gift if it had cleared up with directed pulses the way my chalazion had? (Would the Greek have celebrated their victory over Troy just as much and for as long had the battle lasted a few weeks and been won without woes? Maybe that rogue, Homer, did know a thing or two about the human condition.) Why had the chalazion cleared up in hours many years earlier when I had no conviction of the efficacy of energy healing? Was it to reveal to me one aspect of the miracle of healing? To encourage me to pursue my work with the limbic-spiritual—to show me the light? Why didn't the pustule clear up when I did have strong conviction about such healing many years later? Was that to reveal to me another dimension of that miracle—that the Healer isn't subordinate to my schedule?

How long will the gift of the pustule keep giving? I wonder each morning.

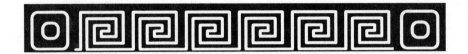

One can only know as much divinity
as exists within one's own self.

Chapter 7

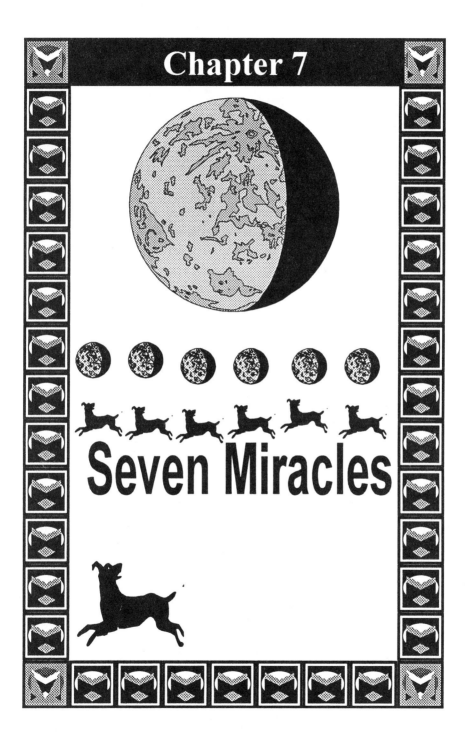

Seven Miracles

I believe in miracles now—I didn't during the 25 years when I practiced mainstream medicine.

I was taught in medical school that miracles are for men of religion, not physicians who practice scientific medicine. For theologists, miracles are events that contradict known scientific knowledge. For lay people, miracles are events that have wondrous consequences but may not be explained or understood. For physicians, miracles are clever deceptions performed by men. Miraclemen, I was further cautioned in medical school, are charlatans from which men of medicine must keep their distance.

As a student, I accepted the party line because I was smug about medicine's scientific foundation—in what I believed was science in medicine. The knowledge that my professors gave I accepted uncritically and mostly mindlessly. Now I have considerable difficulty understanding what scientific knowledge in medicine is and what it isn't.

I have studied medicine for about 40 years. During that time I have read thousands of medical reports discussing great breakthroughs in the drug treatment of immune, degenerative and nutritional disorders. Today we still do not have a single drug that directly repairs damaged antioxidant enzyme systems or reverses chronic degenerative disorders. The scientific "facts" in medicine change daily. Medical journals are replete with *facts* that are subsequently proven false. In fact, more than one dean of medical school has ruefully told the graduating class that 50 percent of what was taught to them in the classroom will be proven wrong with time and that he doesn't know which 50 percent will be proven wrong.

I could cite many examples to explain why I can't be

certain of much of the medical knowledge that is proclaimed to be scientific. What I do know well is that when a safe, nontoxic, nonmutilating therapy relieves suffering for most victims of an illness, it is worth trying. And if such empirical observations are dismissed by some as anecdotes not worthy of the scientists in medicine, so be it!

There is much excitement in the world of physics about predictability and randomness in nature. I am content in letting physicists decide where order in the physical aspects of matter ends and disorder—chaos, as they call it—begins. Until they reach a universal agreement on this most fundamental of all issues in science, I will continue to be guided by empiricism in medicine—namely, what works and is safe in caring for the sick. I am comfortable with ignoring the "science" in drug medicine that suppresses symptoms for some time but leaves sick people sicker and with adverse effects in the long run.

The word miracle also has another meaning: a wondrous happening or a marvelous circumstance; as in, 'She is a miracle of fortitude.' Or as in, 'He made a miraculous recovery.' I prefer this definition of miracle in my clinical work because it allows me to put my clinical observations in a proper frame of reference. I believe a miracle occurs when unrelenting suffering, caused by a chronic disorder, is eased by safe, nontoxic therapies and self-regulation in ways that cannot be explained now by our limited understanding of the healing phenomenon. It is a simple matter of observation, and true observation for me is the purest of all sciences.

There are clearly some observable aspects of healing. I have studied such phenomena with a microscope for almost four decades. I must admit that the essence of the healing process eludes me and my colleagues in pathology alike.

It fascinates me how readily lay people accept the role of hope and spirituality in healing and how resistant to such notions are the majority of physicians. When people outside medicine observe unusual examples of healing, they are excited by such events. When physicians witness a healing they cannot attribute to drugs or scalpels, they are dismayed. Why is it so? This is an important question for us physicians to ponder. Is it because we consider subjects of hope and spirituality threats to our authority? Is it because we see all nondrug and nonscalpel therapies as encroachments on our turf? Or is it that we consider them a threat to our livelihood? Either way, it is unfortunate. Why should it matter to us whether we alleviate a patient's suffering with an herb or a drug? Our professional fees remain the same. Why should we find the efficacy of nutrient injections for promoting recovery from viral infections disconcerting? The compensation for our clinical experience is unaffected whether we administer a vitamin injection or an antibiotic injection. Clearly, nutrient and herbal therapies carry a much larger margin of safety than do drugs.

Medicine is not science. It is the artful application of some aspects of human biology to the care of the sick. The application of the knowledge of physics and chemistry to human suffering is confounded by one essential factor: the human spirit.

The more clinical work I do with patients who have

devastating conditions, such as paralyzing chronic fatigue, multiple sclerosis, AIDS, and cancer, the more I realize the enormous healing power of hope and spirituality supported by therapies proven safe and nontoxic by long empirical experience. And I am increasingly disappointed with the fixed notions of my colleagues in mainstream medicine who think all therapies that do not include drugs or surgical scalpels are quackery.

Who more than physicians should understand the complexity of human systems? Yet, while engineers know how dramatically as few as five variables in a system can affect the output even though the input remains the same, physicians seem not to understand this basic concept of system dynamics. We continue to expect that a given drug will have the same effects on everyone, regardless of different genetic makeups, different biologic burdens, and different emotional and mental states. This notion, in my view, is the main roadblock in understanding the principles and practice of empirical medicine using natural, nondrug therapies.

The debate about psychosomatic and somatopsychic models of disease, as I wrote in *The Cortical Monkey and Healing,* is frivolous. The human condition is a mind-body-spirit continuum.

It is illogical to attempt to separate states produced by the impact of the mind on body tissues from those in which the mind suffers from injured tissues. Such reductionistic thinking—while it may comfort those who thrive on disease classification—is of no concern to serious students of medicine.

Psychosomatic and somatopsychic models of disease are artifacts of thinking. Diseases are caused by burdens on our internal and external environments.

In this chapter I relate some case histories that would be considered miracles by some. Others may choose to dismiss them as "religious" experiences unworthy of medical science. What is important to me is that these case histories represent the truth as I observed it or as it was related to me by my patients. The best part of these miracles is the hope they carry for others with unremitting suffering.

The First Miracle:
A varicose ulcer heals, then cellulitis clears up.

John Y. consulted me for a severe case of varicose veins. His left leg showed a large area of dusky red discoloration with a central area of skin breakdown and ulceration. John had been advised to undergo surgery to remove the varicose veins. John was not ready for surgery and wanted to know if there were any alternatives. John also suffered from many allergies.

Varicose veins are swollen, dilated, and tortuous. The blood stagnates in these veins, obstructing the flow of the fresh blood with oxygen and nutrients into the tissues close to these dilated veins. Deprived of its nourishment, the skin over the dilated varicose veins thins out, sloughs off, and eventually a skin ulcer is formed. Surgery for removal of varicose veins temporarily restores good circulation to the skin and allows the skin ulcer to heal. However, surgery cannot correct the basic weakness in the vein wall structure. Varicose veins often recur, and so do the varicose leg ulcers caused by them.

I explained to John how treatment of allergies and the use of appropriate nutritional protocols could be expected to significantly improve his general circulation and indirectly relieve his varicose veins. I also suggested autoregulation. Specifically, we discussed how John could selectively increase the blood flow through his affected veins and promote healing of the varicose ulcer on his leg. John agreed to follow the autoregulation approach.

I proceeded with a complete physical examination, appropriate blood tests for allergy diagnosis, and suitable nutritional protocols. Following diagnosis of his food and mold allergies, I started an allergy desensitization treatment. At the same time, I started giving John instructions in the principles of autoregulation and methods for facilitating the natural healing responses. The method of directed pulses evidently was most suited for John. So my focus during our training session was on the circulatory aspects.

John turned out to be a natural "autoregger." In the second laboratory session, John told me he was able to bring the pulses to his fingertips, then move them to the ulcerated area of his leg. First he felt tingling in his leg tissues. A few moments later, he felt the pulses. I asked John to do autoregulation for two to fifteen minutes twice a day, and also practice minute-reg (autoregulation done for a minute or two at a time) with a focus on the pulses in the ulcerated area. I make some additional comments about minute-reg in the preceding chapter.

John healed his leg ulcer in seven weeks.

JOHN'S CELLULITIS

About a year later, John came to see me with cellulitis of his right hand and wrist. Cellulitis is a spreading infection of the soft tissues. It causes the tissues to become red, tender, and indurated. Cellulitis is a dangerous infection because it often spreads to the lymphatic channels, then to the bloodstream, resulting in septicemia, a life-threatening emergency. Unless treated aggressively, septicemia produces abscesses in different body tissues and proves fatal.

The skin and tissues involved in cellulitis measured four and a half inches. John's tissues showed no evidence that cellulitis had spread to the area's lymphatics. I drew a blood sample for a blood culture and wrote him a prescription for a broad-spectrum antibiotic.

John had suffered cellulitis of his hand on two previous occasions when he required extended intravenous broad-spectrum antibiotic therapy. During one episode, he was hospitalized for such therapy. Most of the patients I have seen with cellulitis, during my years in surgery, required massive antibiotic therapy in a similar fashion.

Since I knew John was a natural autoregger, I wondered if the same approach would resolve his hand cellulitis. Uncertain of the outcome of such an approach, and with some hesitation, I broached the subject. I fully explained to John the risks of cellulitis, then raised the possibility of controlling that infection with directed pulses. I also explained to him how I was going to monitor the situation closely and would institute antibiotic therapy immediately if I felt we were losing ground. John listened to me carefully, then smiled and told me to proceed. He further told me that he understood both the risks of taking that approach as well as those of massive broad-spectrum antibiotics.

For about 20 minutes, John and I practiced directed pulses. Before he left, I told him to contact me immediately if he developed red streaks (evidence of infection spreading along the lymphatic channels) on his forearm, upper arm, or armpit. I emphasized the importance of not ignoring chills (evidence of bacteria multiplying rapidly in the blood [septicemia]). Finally, I asked John to conduct directed pulses for 10 minutes every hour and to return for a checkup the following day.

When I saw him the next day, the painful, red swelling in the tissues of his right hand was dramatically reduced. I checked to see if there was any evidence of infection spreading along the lymphatic channels, and I found none. Then I asked John to continue practicing directed pulses intermittently and return for a quick visit the following day. There was no sign of cellulitis at all.

It has been more than eight years since I first saw John. He has not had a recurrence of his varicose ulcer nor has he suffered from cellulitis.

The Second Miracle:
An overactive thyroid settles down;
an underactive gland revs up.

Kathy R. consulted me for hyperthyroidism (an overactive thyroid gland) with heart palpitations, hot flushes, excessive sweating, and bouts of anxiety. Her thyroid laboratory tests clearly indicated hyperactivity. Her T_4 test showed an abnormally elevated result. Her doctor had told her that her thyroid problem was most likely caused by an autoimmune disorder—a disorder in which the body's immune defense system turns against its own tissues, the thyroid gland being the target organ in this case. As for treatment, her primary physician referred her to a surgeon, who recommended removal of the overactive gland. She sought a second opinion and was offered alternative treatments of radioactive iodine and drugs. In all cases she was told the result would be the same: a total destruction of the thyroid gland.

Kathy had strong feelings against surgery and radioactive iodine treatment. She was also resistant to the idea of drug therapy for a long period, possibly for several years. She was repulsed by the idea that all three types of treatment were designed to permanently destroy the thyroid gland. She had read quite a bit about the natural healing methods of various cultures and wanted to know if I could guide her in a natural healing effort. Kathy fully understood what she was asking me to do. The physicians she saw previously had given her detailed information about the risks of an overactive thyroid gland, such as heart palpitations and failure, and the probable outcome of untreated hyperthyroidism—a burned-out gland that is functionally useless.

"Do you agree with my previous doctors' diagnoses that thyroid gland overactivity results from an immune injury?" she asked.

"Yes, I do," I replied.

"If this is so, don't you think there might be a way to repair the immune injury?" she continued.

"Probably."

"If that can be done, wouldn't I save my thyroid gland?"

"Probably."

"Don't you think my thyroid gland is worth saving?" she asked with a smile.

"Certainly, it is," I returned her smile.

"So why not try it?"

"We can try, but I don't know if we will succeed. To my knowledge it has never been done. Or rather, it has never been reported in medical literature," I explained.

"That doesn't mean it cannot work, does it?"

"No."

"So why not try it?"

"Well, it's not that simple. There are some ethical and legal issues."

"Dr. Ali, I'll sign any consent you want me to sign. If we fail, I won't hold you responsible. I don't have any alternatives. Will you try? That's all I can ask you," she pleaded, then repeated. "Would you please try?"

Kathy seemed an ideal candidate for a self-regulatory approach. She was evidently quite committed to the idea and was willing to make a diligent attempt at it. Still, it was a difficult decision for me to agree to work with her, fully recognizing the risks involved with untreated hyperthyroidism. After long discussions on two different visits, we decided to proceed.

This was early in my clinical work with natural therapies. My ideas of energetic-molecular medicine, which I describe at length in *RDA: Rats, Drugs and Assumptions*, had not yet evolved. I had no experience dealing with such an "organic" disease using a self-regulatory healing approach. Nobody, to my knowledge, had ever considered hyperthyroidism a psychosomatic disease. At this early stage, I still believed in the distinction between psychosomatic disease (derangement of the mind causing a disease of the body) and somatopsychic disorders (disease of the body causing a derangement of the mind).

Kathy and I began with my nutritional protocols. I asked her to stay on the Tapazole (a drug that destroys an overactive thyroid gland) prescribed by her previous physician. Next, I instructed her in autoregulation methods. The pulses came to her fingertips readily. Within a few days, she learned to direct them to her thyroid gland. I expected this, in a way. An overactive thyroid gland is a rich vascular organ.

Next, I designed a card for Kathy. It showed a microscopic picture of a normal thyroid gland juxtaposed to one displaying the mushroom-like growth of the abnormal cells seen in hyperthyroidism. I asked her to look at this card several times a day. My purpose was to give her true-to-life microscopic imaging for her thyroid gland. I wanted to let her see how her thyroid gland looked in disease and to let her imagine how it would look after she restored it to health.

Kathy, like John, turned out to be a natural autoregger. As she learned to control her symptoms with autoreg, I started reducing the dose of Tapazole. Four months later, Kathy stopped taking Tapazole altogether. Her symptom control with autoreg was complete. Three months later, her thyroid laboratory test results fell from abnormally high values to those within normal range. (T_4 test value fell from 16.8 to 11.4, T_3 value fell from 289 to 156, FTI value fell from 5.1 to 3.4, and T_3 uptake value fell from 34 to 31.)

About 18 months later, Kathy's symptoms recurred. Her laboratory tests became abnormal again. She told me she had taken her prescribed nutrient intermittently and admitted she had stopped doing autoreg. I gave her the choice between Tapazole and autoregulation with nutritional therapies. She chose the autoregulation approach for the second time. About three months later, the symptoms of an overactive thyroid gland had subsided and the results of her thyroid function tests had returned to normal limits. About two years later, her hyperthyroidism recurred for the second time. Again, we began our nondrug program and controlled the overactivity of the gland in some months.

It has been more than three years since the second relapse. She has been free of symptoms and free of drugs. She controls her occasional symptoms with autoregulation without any difficulty, and her high laboratory test values continued gradually to return to the normal range.

One may be tempted to complain about the need for nutrient therapies and autoregulation for so long. Let's look at the alternatives. Almost all patients treated with drugs, surgery, or radioactive iodine for this disorder end up with an underactive thyroid gland (hypothyroidism). Then they have to take thyroid replacement hormones for life. Such therapy requires life-long monitoring for hormone balancing and causes osteoporosis in some cases.

There is another issue of critical importance here. People who develop one type of autoimmune disorder are more likely to develop other types of immune disorders as well. Hyperthyroidism is not an exception. Burning down the thyroid gland with radiation, destroying the gland with chemicals, or removing it with surgery does not address the underlying immune weakness. By contrast, when an overactive thyroid gland is coaxed back to normal behavior with self-regulation, nutrient therapies, and allergy treatment, the weakened immune system is strengthened—not just to cope with an overactive thyroid gland but also to prevent the development of other types of immune disorders.

RADIOACTIVE THERAPY FOR AN 82-YEAR-OLD

How often can one hope to succeed with natural restorative therapies in cases of hyperthyroidism? I have seen only two failures. An 82-year-old woman consulted me for an overactive thyroid gland associated with severe osteoporosis as well as congestive heart failure. She and her husband were very eager to avoid the recommended radioactive iodine treatment. Within days of beginning my nondrug program, I recognized that we didn't have sufficient time to pursue a natural approach. Her heart had been weakened, and I feared that she might slip into a life-threatening, acute heart failure. I recommended radioactive treatment. I didn't get any follow-up from her or her family after that.

The second case concerned a woman in her early forties. After a few weeks of following our program, her primary physician and her husband coerced her into accepting radioactive treatment, and she had her thyroid gland burned down permanently.

A SLUGGISH THYROID GLAND SPEEDS UP

Allan, a man in his late seventies from Boston, consulted me for symptoms of chronic fatigue, allergies, low body temperature, and cold hands and feet. After a clinical laboratory evaluation, I started our nondrug therapies for allergy treatment and prescribed some intramuscular vitamin injections. Because his son practices medicine in Boston, Allan reassured me he would continue the injection therapy suggested. His morning oral temperatures ranged from 96.5 to 97.4. His blood levels of thyroid hormones and TSH test showed evidence of an underactive thyroid gland. I prescribed a small dose of natural thyroid extract. I also incorporated autoregulation, teaching him how to direct his pulses from his fingers to his thyroid gland region, and explained how it was likely to help. He showed good tissue responses in his biologic profile on the computer screen during autoregulation training.

Allan responded well and described a good clinical response during a follow-up phone consultation. At the six-month follow-up he was still doing well. At this time I learned that he had elected not to take the natural thyroid gland extract for some months while he explored the intriguing possibility that he might be able to up-regulate his depressed thyroid gland function with autoreg. My curiosity piqued, and I asked what temperature he was running at that time. He replied:

It's almost one degree higher than it used to be. Directing pulses to my thyroid gland seems like a simple thing to me. Why take a drug unless I have to?

I agreed that it was a good decision on his part and that he should keep a close watch on his body temperature.

It is now more than two and half years since that conversation. He calls infrequently and, at the time of his last call, he still wasn't taking any thyroid gland medication.

Why do the pulses speed up a sluggish thyroid in some patients and not in others? How the body responds to self-regulation depends on several things. First and foremost, there is the issue of total biologic burden: How many diseases is a person fighting? Allen's life has not been unkind to him. He has a loving, supportive wife. His general health was good, except for some undue weakness. He was at peace with himself and with the world around him. He didn't seem to carry hidden anger. Anger, as I wrote in *The Cortical Monkey and Healing,* is the sworn enemy of self-regulation.

There is another important aspect of self-regulation: Angry tissues are impervious to intellectual pleas for healing. Some people have an intuitive sense of how tissues under duress respond to autoregulation, while others stay trapped in cortical devices of mind-over-body healing notions that never work.

Over the years, I have been amazed at the ability of some

people to resolve serious medical problems with little effort in just a few weeks. Equally amazing has been my observation of how some people are so incarcerated in their mind-over-body notions that *repeated pleas from their clever-thinking minds fall on the "deaf ears" of their injured tissues.* On a positive note, nearly all individuals finally do succeed in self-regulation to varying degrees, sometimes after months of struggle. The difference is only a matter of time.

The Third Miracle:
Arthritis in the knee heals with energy.

Irene Q. consulted me for painful swelling in her right knee. She thought her troubles started with a missed step while walking downstairs several months earlier. X-rays showed early stages of arthritis. Several laboratory tests showed negative results. Knee exercises and manipulations gave only temporary relief, and her knee remained swollen. Irene also suffered from other health problems, among them fatigue, recurrent sinusitis, and frequent headaches. She considered herself a "very tense person."

Arthritis is a painful inflammation of the synovium—a thin layer of tissue that lines the joints. The inflamed and swollen synovium begins to erode the joint cartilage. Loss of cartilage first bares and then destroys the underlying bone. The muscles surrounding the joint are irritated and go into spasms to minimize further trauma to the inflamed, sensitive tissues of the synovium, cartilage and bone. The muscle spasm compounds the problem in two ways:

1. It increases mechanical tension on inflamed tissues.
2. It clamps the arteries, reducing the supply of blood to the joint tissues.

These mechanisms feed upon each other and worsen the joint swelling, causing more and more pain, stiffness and swelling.

There are three principal ways that pulses help heal arthritis:

1.   They relax muscles.
2.   They improve circulation and thereby increase the supply of healing nutrients.
3.   They enhance energy dynamics that free musculoskeletal restrictions.

Bone rubbing down bone, that is the core problem of arthritis. This bone-on-bone friction of inflamed joints is worsened as the spastic muscles cause wrenching motions of opposing bone surfaces. What are needed for relief and to promote the healing process are some effective methods of muscle relaxation and improved circulation. Nothing comes close to autoregulation for efficacy.

All tissue healing requires an ample blood supply. When muscles surrounding an inflamed joint are provoked into unrelenting spasms, they literally clamp the arteries going into the joint and drastically reduce the supply of fresh blood to the joint.

Irene responded well to nondrug therapies. Next, I focused on her swollen knee. Specifically, I taught her how to feel pulses in her fingertips. Unlike John and Kathy, it took Irene several weeks to bring clear, strong pulses to her fingertips. But once she succeeded, she learned to direct pulses to her right knee quickly and consistently.

Irene practiced autoregulation religiously. On a follow-up visit three weeks later she told me she had very little pain. The swelling in the knee was gone. But when I saw Irene several weeks later. She told me her pain had returned. The knee was also swollen, though not to the same degree as before. She also told me she had stopped practicing autoregulation after the pain subsided.

I saw Irene four months later. Her face glowed with success. Proudly she told me how she had controlled the pain and swelling with autoregulation. Even her fellow teachers noticed how she was able to walk down the stairs pain-free, without any limp. She said,

I have learned my lesson. I don't dare skip my autoreg now.

Pain and other symptoms are barometers of biology. They are clarion calls for relief from a biology under stress. We can hear these calls, respond with a timeout, and remove the stressor. Or we can dull the signal from biology with drugs. That is a clear choice. Irene and Kathy were among the first to give me this important insight.

The concept of natural energy dynamics in the human body, as I wrote earlier, may be unsettling to those who have never engaged in tissue energy work. But the concept is readily understood by meditators and my patients during autoregulation training. Autoregulation dramatically improves subtle energies in inflamed joint tissues and promotes natural healing responses.

The Fourth Miracle:
A concrete slab in the chest melts away.

Alice Y., a women in her late forties, was referred to me by her physician for a chronic illness caused by exposure to industrial chemicals, including halogenated compounds and some toxic compounds of nickel, mercury, cadmium and lead. For many years she had worked in a chemical factory. Her illness included severe fatigue, palpitations, wild mood swings, inability to concentrate, frequent throat and respiratory infections, sinus pressure with headaches and skin bruises. As is the case in most patients with chemical sensitivity, Alice also suffered from mold and pollen allergy.

A few weeks before Alice saw me, she was admitted to a hospital with chest pains. A heart attack was suspected. She had been under severe and unrelenting stress. She looked dejected and in despair. Chemically sensitive patients often tolerate prescription drugs poorly. This was true of Alice. She knew the answer to her illness could not be drugs. She said, "I'm carrying a slab in my chest."

Alice felt much stronger within weeks of starting our management plan, and many of her symptoms subsided. But she obtained no relief from her main symptom—that 'slab-in-the-chest' sensation.

At this time I was beginning to understand the value of the directed pulses. So I decided to shift my focus to this technique.

I taught Alice the principles and practice of autoregulation and prepared an autoregulation tape for her. I taught her how to bring the pulses to her fingertips then transfer those pulses to her shoulder, neck and chest areas. On a follow-up visit two weeks later, I was surprised to hear Alice was able to dissolve the concrete slab. Alice continued to suffer from stress, anxiety and palpitations off and on for the next several months. On some bad days, the slab would return. But there was a difference now. She now had control over the concrete slab. On a follow-up visit, she said,

Autoreg is my drug now. This drug has no side effects.

As with many other patients, autoregulation became a part of Alice's life.

Nearly eight years have passed since my initial work with Alice. Her symptom of the slab in chest returned from time to time during the first few years which she usually controlled with autoregulation. Once she came down with *H. pylori* infection of the stomach, for which she was given massive doses of antibiotics by other physicians (not a good plan of therapy for *H. pylori*, in my view). Antibiotic therapy caused a relapse of many other symptoms, including extreme stress, heart palpitations, and the slab in her chest. At that time she couldn't control her symptoms with autoregulation, and I had to prescribe small doses of Ativan. Several months later, the trauma of undergoing foot surgery caused a full-blown relapse of all her original symptoms including the slab in the chest. Again, she required small doses of antianxiety medication. Some months later, Alice's *H. pylori*-related symptoms returned and a stomach biopsy showed the microbes. This time she opted for my nondrug plan of therapy rather than take heavy doses of Flagyl and other antibiotics. She recovered nicely with nutrient and herbal therapies and without antibiotics.

(*H. pylori* can never be permanently banished from the stomach with drugs. The real issue in this infection is the integrity of the stomach ecosystem. Microbes do not make homes in stomachs that are healthy. The *H. pylori* organism flourishes in the stomach only when the gastric ecology is damaged by stomach acidity disorders, antacid abuse, oxidized and denatured foods, stress of modern life, and by events that disrupt a normal bowel ecosystem.)

At the time of this writing, Alice has experienced neither the symptoms of heart palpitations and the slab in the chest nor of *H. pylori* gastritis for over three years. I relate her case history for a very important reason: Complete resolution of health problems with nondrug therapies and autoregulation is at times maddeningly slow. Yet, the long-term results make the efforts worthwhile.

The Fifth Miracle:
Cystitis clears up with pulses.

Some people are incredibly intuitive. Susan C. turned out to be one such patient.

In her early forties, Susan saw me for chronic urinary difficulties. Strangely, she had considerable difficulty voiding at home and wasn't able to urinate at all in public restrooms. Urine cultures had been consistently negative. Repeated courses of antibiotics and Nystatin, prescribed on the assumption that her urinary symptoms might have been due to occult bladder infection or possibly *Candida* yeast overgrowth, hadn't helped. On three separate occasions, Susan's urologist tried to address the problem with urethral dilatations under anesthesia. The urologist hoped that, once stretched, the muscle in the region of the neck of the urinary bladder would remain loose and relieve her symptoms. All three attempts failed.

Susan hoped that perhaps I could mitigate her problem by detecting and treating hidden food and mold allergies. She attended my autoregulation class before the laboratory test results became available for review. She became intrigued with the possibility of improving her bladder sphincter function with autoreg, especially with directed pulses to the urethral opening.

As it turned out, Susan was another natural autoregger. During the next visit, even before I could suggest that she try directed pulses to control her bladder symptoms, she told me she had gotten the idea of doing so during my autoreg workshop and that she had learned to direct pulses to her bladder sphincter (about an inch below and deep to the pubic bone). Furthermore, she was excited about the initial positive response to directed pulses. I was happy to learn of her initial experiment and made some further suggestions.

At a follow-up visit six weeks later, Susan said,

This stuff is science fiction—too good to believe! I have suffered from painful urination for years. I have had cystoscopies and urethral dilatations done. I have taken antibiotics so many times. My doctor tried Nystatin several times. And now this. I bring pulses to my sphincter and I am able to go. God, it is that simple. Who would believe it?

Susan visited me on a few occasions after she made the above comment and reported continued relief from her urinary symptoms. Then I didn't see her for some years. I wondered whether the benefits of autoregulation had lasted or whether they had simply faded away.

One day while writing this chapter—about six years after my initial consultation with Susan—I asked some nurses if anyone remembered her and had heard any further follow-up information about her bladder problems. A nurse looked at me curiously, then asked why I questioned her on that particular day. I told her I was working on my autoregulation book and my thoughts just happened to wander to Susan's bladder problems. She laughed, asked me to wait, and stepped out of the office. Moments later, the nurse returned with a man. "This is Susan's husband," she grinned. "He comes here sometimes to pick up nutrient protocols you prescribed for Susan."

I asked Susan's husband some general questions about Susan, then inquired about Susan's bladder sphincter function. He replied,

Doctor Ali, we still laugh at that sometimes. If that isn't a miracle, I don't know what is. She has been free of her bladder symptoms ever since she learned to direct her pulses to her bladder sphincter. No more anesthesia! No more cystoscopies! No more urethral dilatation. Unbelievable, isn't it?

I don't witness such healing often. But when it does happen, it restores my faith in the unfathomable wisdom of body tissues—and in miracles.

The Sixth Miracle:
Pulses open the bronchial tubes.

When I returned to clinical medicine after more than 20 years of research and practice in pathology, I developed a working definition of empirical medicine that held the following four elements important:

1. I should use therapies that work.
2. I should use therapies that are free of long-term toxicities.
3. I should not let discussions about the mechanisms of action cloud my judgment.
4. I should dismiss as irrelevant all prognostications based on published controlled and blinded drug studies and recognize that *the only true control for evaluating a clinical outcome for an individual is himself or herself.*

I was comfortable with the use of microscopes and laboratory tests as far as science in medicine was concerned. In my clinical practice I wanted to focus on how I could integrate natural therapies that have been proven safe and effective by empirical observations for centuries in my management plan. Furthermore, I needed to know how I could enhance their clinical value with oral and injectable nutrient protocols that I was using for clinical research. I didn't want frivolous notions of double-blind cross-over studies to distract me. I discuss this subject at length and support my viewpoint with extensive reviews of literature in the companion volume *RDA: Rats, Drugs and Assumptions.*

There are special rewards for physicians who will not let themselves be governed by medical texts. Craig A. was the first of my many patients who helped me realize some of those rewards.

A police officer in his early thirties, Craig had been treated for asthma for several years with inhalers, theophylline, anti-histamines and steroids. Still, he suffered eight to ten asthma attacks a day. At 15, he had developed irregular heartbeats and was diagnosed with Wolff-Parkinson-White syndrome, a type of heart disease that causes arrhythmias (irregular heartbeats) and can be fatal. He was put on quinidine for his heart disorder.

In addition, Craig had multiple pollen, mold and food allergies. He was also sensitive to environmental pollution. I treated his allergies and chemical sensitivities with my allergy and nutritional protocols. Five months after Craig first saw me, his asthma was controlled without drugs. Then I decided to desensitize him to foods—an approach that, contrary to prevailing notions of drug medicine in the United States, sometimes does work well. I realized this could bring Craig's asthma back temporarily, so I explained that possibility to him and prepared him for that possibility by teaching autoregulation.

Craig received his first food desensitization injection in the afternoon and woke up that night with an asthma attack. In my experience, such delayed reactions to desensitization injections are not uncommon during the initial desensitization period, but are extremely rare later on. He called me the following morning and said,

An asthma attack woke me at about three a.m. I did some autoreg. I brought pulses to my fingertips and that was it. My asthma attack was under control. I didn't have to use my inhaler or other medication. I just went back to sleep.

A few months after Craig learned to control his asthma with autoregulation, I reduced the dose of his heart medication and discontinued it altogether several weeks later. Craig remained free of asthma and all asthma drugs for more than 29 months after he learned to control his bronchial spasms with nondrug therapies. Nor did he suffer from episodes of irregular heartbeats. Management of food allergy cured him of his Wolff-Parkinson-White (WPW) syndrome—a potentially fatal disease that he never had. (I wonder how many other Craigs there are living in fear of sudden death from WPW whose cardiac arrhythmias are triggered by undiagnosed food allergies.)

Bronchospasm—an asthma attack in lay terms—is often triggered by stress and is highly responsive to effective self-regulatory methods. Each asthma patient needs to learn such methods. Even when steroid abuse rules out the kind of results Craig enjoyed, an asthmatic can dramatically reduce the dosage of drugs for asthma control. There have been no exceptions in my practice.

As a safety measure, asthmatics should always have easy access to asthma drugs for times when multiple exposures to environmental chemicals and molds provoke an intense asthma attack. This also holds for asthmatics who experience excellent control with nondrug therapies.

I discuss some essential issues in the nondrug management of asthma in *The Cortical Monkey and Healing*. Here, I wish to emphasize one simple and often effective natural therapy that may help control an asthma attack: Drink four liters of water with one-half to one teaspoon of sea salt. Again, asthma attacks can prove dangerous and should be managed under close supervision of an experienced physician.

The Seventh Miracle:
Pulses clear up hives.

David Z., a nine-year-old hyperactive boy, was brought to see me by his parents, who were at their wits' end. He suffered from constant hives caused by food and mold allergies. His other symptoms included wild mood swings and a short attention span. The professional staff at his school had diagnosed him as "perceptually impaired." Blood tests showed very high levels of IgE antibodies (antibodies that cause common pollen and mold allergies and some forms of food allergy).

I treated David with the appropriate allergy and nutritional protocols and taught him how to do pulses. On one visit, I taught him autoregulation and showed him a graph of his pulses, heart activity, and electrical impulses in his skin and muscles on the computer screen. The graphs demonstrated wild fluctuations before and smooth and even lines after he directed pulses to his fingertips. David was visibly excited by what he considered a computer game.

Beaming with evident satisfaction, David said,

I got pulses in my fingertips. I also got them in my ears.

David's hives are under control now, except on days when

he is exposed to large quantities of pollen and molds. Here are some comments David's father made during a follow-up visit:

David controls the hives completely with autoreg when he wants to. But you know he is a boy and sometimes doesn't have the patience for it. Still, it is a far cry from the way things were. Now we know we can control it if we have to.

I might relate here David's father's experience with choices in the kitchen, which I recommended for David. I advise parents of food-allergic children to make the necessary changes in food selection for the entire family rather than cook separately for their allergic child. For David, I excluded dairy as well as beef. After several days of avoiding beef himself, David's father observed his elevated values of systolic and diastolic blood pressure gradually come down. I should add here that I do not often see such dramatic responses in blood pressure to changing choices in the kitchen.

Children learn self-regulation well. Understandably, they often lack the patience and perseverance to practice self-regulation frequently. However, whenever I have been able to persuade them to learn autoregulation, the results have been gratifying. Frequently, I ask parents to learn some methods of autoregulation and make a game of it to play with the child. In some cases of attention deficit disorder and hyperactivity, limbic breathing has been especially valuable as a part of our total program emphasizing nutrient therapies and allergy treatment. The same holds for some cases of autism, Tourette's syndrome, and children with developmental problems.

Below, I reproduce two pages of text from the forthcoming volume, *Lata, Limbic Breathing and Healing*. Limbic breathing is an autoregulation method I teach my patients in order to facilitate a healing response.

LIMBIC BREATHING FOR CHILDREN

Sandra was only 19 months old when she learned to control some of her asthma with limbic breathing.

Sandra suffered from food allergy soon after she was born. She developed full-blown asthma attacks before she reached her first birthday. She was on regular doses of theophylline (a broncho-dilator drug used for asthma control) and additionally required multiple daily doses of another inhaler medication to control asthma attacks. Like most other children with asthma, Sandra developed frequent infections and had been treated with antibiotics on several occasions.

After making the diagnosis of food, mold, and pollen allergies with micro-ELISA blood tests, I put Sandra on our allergy desensitization and nutritional protocols. I also excluded certain food items from her diet. As the frequency and intensity of her asthma attacks diminished, I gradually reduced the dose of her drugs. After 13 weeks, Sandra's asthmatic symptoms were completely relieved, and I discontinued all drugs.

I knew that complete control of asthma without drugs requires success in all three approaches of energetic-molecular medicine: allergy, nutrition and self-regulation. Every time I saw Sandra in our office for an allergy injection, I tried to think of a method for teaching Sandra autoregulation. Each time I drew a blank. She was obviously too young to be engaged in a discussion on my concepts of how the cortical monkey causes diseases, and how limbic-spiritual healing occurs. It was obvious that I could not explain to her how her bronchi (air tubes) tightened to cause asthma attacks, and how she could loosen them with autoregulation to ease her breathing. I had to improvise.

Sandra's mother often brought her two older children to the office. They would play with Sandra as if she was their doll. One day I saw them hold Sandra by her arms and lift her up with swinging movements. That opened a window for me.

Since I cannot explain to Sandra how to direct healing energy to her bronchi, what if I taught her how to direct it to some other part of her body? What if she could learn to be aware of that body organ? What if I then taught her how to "transfer" that awareness to her bronchial tubes?

I recognized I could not relate to Sandra at an intellectual level. But perhaps that was not necessary. Her older brother and sister, at a level Sandra well understood, related to her quite well. Perhaps I could reach Sandra through her siblings.

I called Sandra's mother to my consultation room where I explained to her how I was going to approach the problem of teaching Sandra autoregulation to normalize her breathing if her asthma recurred. I told Sandra's mom to start playing a "limbic game" at home with Sandra and her other two children. In this game, they will stand in a circle, half stretch their arms, and hold each others hands. Then they will raise their hands gradually and gently breathe in for three seconds (the breathe-in), keep their hands up for two seconds (the hold period), then very evenly and slowly breathe out for four to six seconds (the breathe-out period). After two or three regular breaths, they will repeat the sequence. I explained to Sandra's mother that this would help Sandra to learn pacing for limbic breathing. It will also seed the core idea of autoregulation in Sandra's mind.

When a person attends to a part of his body, it responds.

After a few weeks passed, Sandra came down with a cold and developed wheezing. That is when Sandra's mother and two siblings tried the limbic game. For the first time, Sandra dissolved her asthma attack without drugs.

In the eighteen months after Sandra first controlled asthma with autoregulation, her mom observed several similar episodes. Of course, on other occasions she required some medication.

Autoregulation comes easier to children. They do not carry any loads of disbelief. They need not unload burdens they do not carry in the first place.

Science in Medicine

Earlier in this chapter, I wrote that many hard-core medical "scientists" scoff at the case histories I use to illustrate the potential benefits of limbic-spiritual healing. I know that my colleagues in mainstream medicine dismiss all nondrug and nonscalpel therapies as unscientific quackery.

But what is science in medicine? First and foremost, true science is purity of observation. An observed episode of healing must not be dismissed just because it does not fit into preconceived notions. I devote the companion volume, *RDA: Rats, Drugs and Assumptions,* to this essential subject. In this volume, I cite three instances of how "scientific" medicine has operated in the past. Those three situations make me wonder how future physicians will regard what we consider science in clinical medicine today.

MEDICAL "SCIENCE" OF GENITAL MUTILATION

In 1861, Isaac Baker Brown, an eminent London surgeon, recommended amputation of the clitoris for the treatment of headaches, PMS symptoms, and mental illness in girls and young women. He claimed to achieve excellent clinical results from this operation and was recognized as a prominent and influential member of the Obstetrical Society. After many years of enjoying great fame and fortune for his surgical prowess, Brown fell in disgrace. Interestingly, Brown wasn't vilified for mutilating the genitals of many girls and young women, but because he angered someone at the Commissioners of Lunacy for unlawfully detaining a young woman with the intent of amputating her clitoris. When public furor forced the London Obstetrical Society to investigate Brown in March 1867 and consider his expulsion, a problem arose: The Society's members couldn't punish Brown for performing a clitoridectomy because they themselves were "clitoridectomists." Finally, on April 3, 1867, the Society voted to expel him—not for performing the operation but for failing to obtain the consent of the patient's family (*Journal of Obstetrics and Gynecology of the British Empire* 67:1017-1034; 1867).

It is unsettling to read accounts of barbaric rituals of genital mutilation among some ancient tribal cultures. Anthropologist Jomo Kenyatta, who later served as the first president of independent Kenya, defended ritual clitoridectomy in tribal Kenya in a book published in the late 1930s. But he seemed very uncomfortable doing so. How does one comprehend medical "science" in blaming the clitoris for headache, PMS symptoms and mental illness in the nineteenth century? How does one understand the barbaric acts of English surgeons who committed heinous crimes of mutilation in the name of medical science?

MEDICAL "SCIENCE" OF DESTROYING THE IMMUNE SYSTEM WITH RADIATION

On August 29, 1994, I saw a C-Span TV program in which a submariner who received radium treatments at age 18, described his case history in a testimony delivered before the Senate

Subcommittee for the Environment chaired by Senator Joseph Lieberman. The submariner's throat was radiated to keep his ears from bleeding during the "tank test"—an exercise in which submarine trainees are required to practice escape techniques in simulated deep water conditions. The submariner developed episodes of voice loss, nasal discomfort, peculiar tooth fractures, and finally came down with cancer of the nasopharynx.

The submariner was radiated by Connecticut M.D., Harry Haines who was a forceful proponent for solving the ear problems of submarine crews with radiation treatments. Emboldened by his experience with submariners, Haines began to radiate the throats, ears, and necks of little children to treat common viral and bacterial infections. Doctors at Johns Hopkins in Baltimore were impressed by the results Haines reported and began to radiate their own pediatric patients, as well as adult patients with similar problems. They also excelled in using radiation to treat acne and the enlarged thymus glands of children and young people. Most of these children grew up with severely damaged immune systems, and many developed cancers of the thyroid gland and other tissues of the head and neck region.

Treating tonsillitis, acne, and thymus enlargement with radiation was considered good *science* in medicine. Whenever I see a patient with a severely damaged immune system resulting from radiation, I wonder how any intelligent physician could be so simple-minded. How is it that Dr. Haines and others at Johns Hopkins did not recognize the widely known dangers of radiation?

One internist at our hospital received radiation treatments for acne of the face and upper torso during childhood. During the 1970s, I diagnosed many cancers in his skin biopsies. The internist grew crops of basal cell cancers in radiated areas of his skin. He was fortunate that his dermatologist watched him closely and removed the skin cancers during early stages. I know of many patients who were not that lucky.

I have seen patients with severe immune problems whose enlarged thymus glands were radiated during childhood—many years after widely publicized reports demonstrated that radiation caused cancers in Japanese children in Hiroshima and Nagasaki. The irony is that an enlarged thymus gland in a child is an innocent condition that causes no problems and, in most cases, is incidentally diagnosed with X-rays taken for unrelated reasons.

MEDICAL "SCIENCE" OF DESTROYING IMMUNE SYSTEMS WITH KILLER DRUGS

I have cared for many young men who were infected with the HIV virus in the early 1980s—long before their partners died of AIDS in the mid-1980s. They are living full, productive lives. Some of them developed lesions of Kaposi's sarcoma (a form of malignant tumor of the blood vessels), *Pneumocystis carinii* and other lung infections and oral ulcers. One young man had malignant melanoma removed on two occasions. The remarkable thing about this group of patients is that none of them took AZT, DDI, DDC, or similar toxic, antiviral drugs. All of them followed broad holistic programs with a focus on nutritional support, herbal and other natural antiviral therapies, meditation and spiritual work. I do not know of any patient who became infected during the early 1980s, who took marrow-killing toxic AIDS drugs unsupported by natural immune-enhancing therapies for more than five years, who is still symptom-free fifteen years later. On many occasions, I have asked for such examples on radio shows. To date, no one has called to tell me of a long-term HIV survivor who accepted toxic drug therapies.

Many studies show that drug therapies do not prolong survival in patients with AIDS. The survival in HIV-positive persons, with or without clinical evidence of AIDS, is vastly improved with natural, nondrug, restorative therapies that support an individual's antioxidant, enzyme and immune defenses.

In a cohort study of 5,833 individuals with AIDS in New York City, survival in HIV-positive gay men was compared with that of HIV-positive African-American and Hispanic women (*N Eng J Med* 317:1297; 1987). After one year, the cumulative probability of survival among men with AIDS was over 80 percent, while that for women was about 30 percent. After two years, the figure for men was over 50 percent, while that for women was about 10 percent. What are the possible reasons for such a wide discrepancy between mortality among men and women that has not been observed in the case of any other virus? The most likely explanation for this difference is that gay men quickly learned aspects of the biology of HIV infection, made the needed lifestyle changes, and had the resources to seek and obtain effective natural, nondrug therapies. The African-American and Hispanic women of New York City were not that lucky. Also, it seems likely that administration of highly toxic drugs for HIV infection, without any efforts to buttress the damaged immune system with nutritional therapies, hastened the death of many women.

"ALL MY FRIENDS DIED WITH AZT; I WONDERED IF I COULD LIVE WITHOUT IT"

David L., an Italian male in his mid-thirties, thinks he was exposed to the HIV virus in 1980 or 1981. Some of his friends developed AIDS and were treated intensively with AZT and other drugs. One by one, they died of AIDS in the early and mid-1980s. David's physicians in Italy advised him to be tested for HIV infection and to undergo drug treatments if the test showed HIV infection. Initially he declined the antibody test. When he was finally tested in 1985, the test confirmed what David already knew. Despite persistent pleading by his physicians, David declined AZT and other drug treatments.

In the summer of 1995, David flew to New York to consult me. I was very curious as to why he had stubbornly declined drug treatment.

"David, why did you refuse treatment?" I asked.

"I didn't refuse treatment," he replied in a thick accent.

"But didn't you just now tell me that you repeatedly refused to take AZT, DDI and related drugs?"

"Yes, I did," he smiled. "I only refused AZT, DDI and other drugs. I didn't say no to other therapies."

"What other therapies?"

"Natural and herbal therapies."

"Who was treating you?" I asked, my curiosity piqued.

"I found some good herbalists and naturopaths." He flashed another smile.

"Oh," I said, trying not to sound surprised, as I studied

David's face for some moments and wondered what I was going to make of the situation. "You are in your mid-thirties now," I began, recovering. "You were in your mid-twenties then. Help me understand how a young man says no to drug treatment for a disease that is considered fatal by everyone."

"It wasn't a difficult decision." David became somber.

"Not difficult?" I asked, incredulous. "What decision can be more important than a life-death decision like that?"

"It wasn't difficult, at least not then," David laughed lightly.

"So?" I pressed.

"There wasn't that much to think about, Dr. Ali," he replied. "All my friends died while taking AZT. I was prepared to die too. But it occurred to me that if I was going to die, I might as well die without AZT. Then I wondered if I could live without it."

"Prepared to die," I murmured to myself, then repeated after him, "die without AZT."

How does a young man learn to talk about death like that? How does he cope with the fear of death? How does he plan for his own imminent death with such serenity? What does he say to his family? Or friends? Or himself? I looked into David's soft blue eyes, looking for answers to my questions. He held my gaze.

"There were circumstances before that, weren't there?" I asked after a while.

"Yes, there were," he replied.

"You don't have to tell me if you don't want," I said reassuringly.

"There is nothing to hide. My brother was also gay. We grew up in a puritan home. Those were difficult times. I knew there had to be answers somewhere. So before the AIDS epidemic started, I found some good teachers and learned to seek spiritual growth. I became a vegetarian and learned to meditate. I think I shed a lot of my anger then. So when the HIV virus hit me and my friends began to die, I delved deeper into spiritual work. AZT simply didn't seem to be the answer for me. I was prepared to die. I didn't know then that I was also prepared to live with the virus."

Until I met David, it had never occurred to me that HIV would change so many lives in utterly unpredictable ways—that for many people, the virus would be a medium for spiritual transcendence. Now that I look back, I ask, Why not? Haven't I seen people for whom cancer has done the same thing? Aren't there hundreds of thousands of people all over the world whose course in life has been forever changed by a malignant tumor?

A POSITIVE HIV TEST: WHAT DOES IT MEAN?

In the early 1980s, I—like my colleagues—looked at HIV as a killer virus. The prevailing pronouncement then was that a positive HIV test indicated an inexorable downhill course that would always end with the patient's demise. I equated signing a positive HIV antibody test report to that of signing a death certificate. Then, as I began to see patients like David with positive tests, I began to question the party line. David taught me to look at the HIV virus—if indeed it exists as a single discrete virus—in an altogether different light.

It seems likely that the HIV-AIDS story will prove to be a monumental tragedy. We "diagnose" HIV infection with antibody tests just as we diagnose rheumatoid arthritis with antibody tests. In both cases, we do not fully know what those antibodies are directed against. In both cases, the detection of antibodies leads to a diagnostic label and dangerous assumptions about the biologic significance of those antibodies. It is a basic premise of immunology that the mere presence of antibodies does not prove anything. It is essential that we characterize what those antibodies are directed against.

After more than 15 years of intensive research at the cost of billions of dollars, the absolute criteria for proving the existence of the HIV virus have yet to be met. There are three essential criteria for establishing the presence of a new virus:

1. Virus particles of the same shape and size should be seen in the infected tissues with an electron microscope;
2. Proteins of the virus coat should be isolated and proven to be unique; and
3. The viral DNA or RNA should be isolated and unequivocally proven to be distinct.

Many experienced virologists question that these essential criteria have been met in the case of HIV. They have growing doubts about many assumptions that have been made about establishing the identity of HIV. Is New York HIV the same as New Dehli HIV? Is an HIV-induced disorder in Moscow identical to that which is seen in the people of Missouri? If HIV is a unique virus, why have all attempts to produce an effective vaccine against it failed? AIDS was described initially as a disease of gay men. Now the highest rate of new cases is among African-American and Hispanic women. What made HIV change its mind?

Widely publicized pictures of the HIV virus are nearly

always captioned as a *virus-like* particle. It seems likely that there is not just one HIV virus, but a family of cousin-viruses produced by rapid mutations. This also explains why all attempts to prepare an effective vaccine to date have failed.

How does a physician use such flimsy evidence to justify annihilating a patient's immune defenses with potent poisons? And to think that some ill-informed politicians are pushing AZT on unborn babies by legally mandating HIV tests on all pregnant women.

The fundamental difference between immune-enhancing and immune-destroying approaches to caring for patients with AIDS emerged during the early years of the epidemic. Gay men, who quickly educated themselves on the syndrome, embarked on holistic programs with nutrients, herbs and meditation, and fared much better than those whose immune systems were further suppressed by highly toxic antiviral drugs.

In its December 28, 1989 issue, *The New England Journal of Medicine* reported that, "the hazard rate for mortality was higher in children receiving the diagnosis early in life....The median survival for all 172 children was 38 months." My interpretation of the *Journal's* data is simple: An infant's immune system is largely a reflection of his mother's immune system during the first months of life. Since the mother's defenses had been shattered with factors that make up AIDS, it is predictable that their babies would have serious difficulties fighting off common viral and bacterial infections. The *Journal*, however, took a different position and advised its readers as follows: "Early diagnosis is important, since there is only a short interval in which to initiate prophylactic or antiviral treatment before progressive disease begins."

What the *Journal* really advocates here is that newborn babies with evidence of the HIV infection should be hit early and hard with drugs used for treating AIDS. What kind of data does the *Journal* have to support the use of drastic, immune-destructive therapies for newborns and toddlers? How long was the follow-up study conducted of newborns and infants who were administered AZT, DDI and related drugs? Was it two years or four? Such studies were initiated only a few years ago. Evidently no one yet knows the long-term devastation on the immune systems of their "research" subjects. I am certain the fate of these infants will be worse than those of children given radiation for tonsillitis, acne and enlarged thymus glands. It will be worse because the long-term consequences of localized radiation are not nearly as horrendous as those caused by immune annihilation.

One generation of medical "researchers" now makes a name for itself by publishing papers extolling the virtues of AIDS drugs for infants. Decades from now—I'm certain—another generation of medical researchers will make a name for itself by publishing reports of strange cancers and immune disorders among infants who now have toxic drugs administered to them.

MEDICAL "SCIENCE" OF IMMUNE DESTRUCTION IN UNBORN BABIES

The case of infants facing a serious disease understandably raises special concerns. People inside and outside medicine feel a greater sense of urgency to do something about the situation. Since immune-enhancing, nondrug therapies are frowned upon in traditional medicine, such concerns inevitably bring forth louder voices for more drug therapies.

The New York Times published an article in its August 3, 1995, issue with the following headline:

SACRIFICING BABIES ON THE ALTER OF PRIVACY

The article reported that some 7,000 babies are born each year in the United States to HIV-infected women, and about 2,000 of the infants test positive for HIV. "Fortunately," it further told its readers, "nearly three quarters of these are false positive, because the babies have their mother's antibodies, but not HIV itself." The article then made an impassioned plea that all pregnant women should have HIV testing done so that the unborn babies can be treated.

The article also referred to legislation introduced by some congressmen that would require testing all newborns whose mothers were not tested for HIV, informing the parents or guardians, and counseling them about the steps necessary to save the lives of their children. Save the lives of the children! But, how? Evidently, those legislators believe the babies should be fed AZT, DDI and related drugs to save them from the virus.

I shuddered when I read the article. Do these legislators have any sense as to how delicate the immune systems of newborns are? Do they know how immune-destructive AZT, DDI and related drugs are? Do they recognize how many severe infections such babies will get after their immune defenses have been destroyed with drugs? How many of the newborns will die of such infections? And how many of those who survive the immediate drug toxicity will live with permanently damaged antioxidant and immune defenses, if they live beyond a decade or two anyway? We know that adults who begin with much stronger immune defenses do not live for more than a few years after taking the drugs. What makes the legislators think the newborns, who are dependent upon the immunity of their mothers, will survive the drug assault any better?

Obviously, the legislators and the writer of the *Times* article are well-intentioned. They are not immunologists. They are not well-informed about true immediate, short- and long-term drug toxicities of the immune-destroying drugs used for HIV. They are making the sad mistake of taking the drug doctors' words as gospel. And physicians who promote those drug therapies say what their paymasters in the drug industry tell them. Natural, immune-enhancing therapies have no constituency.

A SAD CHAPTER IN THE HISTORY OF MEDICINE

I'm afraid that when the history of twentieth-century medicine is written, the use of toxic, immune-destructive drugs for HIV infection unsupported by immune-enhancing therapies will be recognized as a dark blotch—a barbaric chemical annihilation of the immune defenses of people who desperately needed restorative therapies. The future physician may well consider our present immune-destroying drug therapies for HIV as abominable as those of genital mutilations on young women for headaches and the radiation of children for tonsillitis by the physicians of yesteryear.

THE SPIRITUAL
AND THE MIND-OVER-BODY DOGMA

David is one of my patients who has helped me understand the hollowness of prevailing dogmas on mind-over-body healing. *It simply does not work.* There are limited benefits to the so-called positive thinking and directed imagery healing. To date, I have not seen long-term success in healing patients with life-threatening disorders, such as AIDS, cancer, and paralyzing multiple sclerosis, with superficial notions. Good long-term results are possible in such disorders only when the patient breaks through the confines of the thinking mind and seeks spiritual enlightenment for its own sake—and not to seek spirituality as a cure for a fatal disease. David did it the right way.

The ancient notion of mind-body-spirit, by definition, holds that the spiritual must be outside the capacity of all physical senses and beyond the reach of the intellect. Evidently, whatever we can perceive with our senses or imagine with our mind falls in the domains of the body and mind. Why come up with the trio of mind-body-spirit if the human condition was limited to intellectual or bodily functions? Why didn't the ancients stop at the duo of mind-body? The spiritual is the unknowable—except through the profound changes it brings in the lives of those who seek it. I have seen patients with cancer undergo profound changes only when they broke through the limits set by the thinking mind. I have seen them lose all their prejudices and become free of distinctions between races, colors, and creeds through deep spiritual work. Yet, none of them could define what the spiritual is. (Nor did they care to do so.) Cancer gave them a true freedom to live a different and much richer life. It is the same with AIDS. That is the message of David's story.

I close this chapter with the following text from *The Cortical Monkey and Healing:*

> *It seems improbable that man will ever fully understand the healing energy of love, or to be more precise, the healing energy of God. Medical technology, itself an expression of God's energy, is beginning to allow us to measure some things about love...One day, it seems, the men of medicine and the men of spirits will meet at some summit of union. The energy of love will have brought them together.*

Spirituality is awareness of the linkage with the presence *that permeates and surrounds each of us without being distressed about what the nature of that linkage might be.*

From *Life, Healing and Thinking Ants*

Water facilitates healing more than any other single healing agent. All wise physicians know that. Water fascinates people more than any other element in nature. Artists and scientists recognize that. How did water achieve such importance? Perhaps because all life on planet Earth crawled out of the primordial oceans.

From *Do Fish Know Water?*

Chapter 8

My
Mistakes

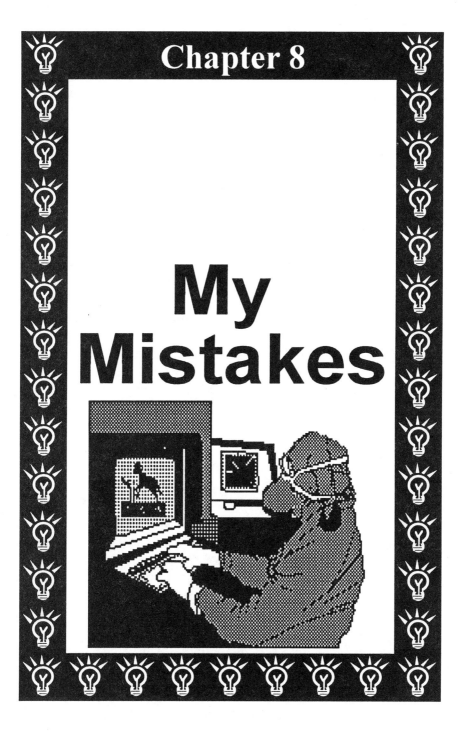

The only way one can completely avoid mistakes is if one makes no decisions at all. Since a physician cannot avoid making decisions, he can only hope that his mistakes are not too frequent, and those he makes are not too dangerous and do not create irreversible consequences. I have made my share of mistakes in my professional work. In this chapter, I describe a few that illustrate some aspects of my work with autoregulation and the limbic-spiritual.

Microscopy has been a consuming passion for about thirty years. As a pathology resident, I threw myself at the microscope with an obsessive-compulsive drive that bordered vengeance (against what I didn't know). I remember that if a slide didn't speak to me right away, I took it as a personal affront. A continuing gift from God to me is that microscopic diagnosis never stressed me during the twenty-nine years I worked as a hospital pathologist. I can say that safely even after carrying the responsibility for diagnosis of more than 40,000 cancers and over 100,000 diagnostic specimens during the last thirty years.

As a young pathologist, my pathology work gave me a sense that if one worked diligently and with discipline, one could succeed in avoiding almost all mistakes. Years later, when I returned to clinical medicine for work in energetic-molecular (EM) medicine, I assumed that I could avoid mistakes by doing diligent, disciplined work in this new medicine as well. I failed to recognize that it had taken me years to learn the safe practice of pathology, and that it was naive to assume that I could achieve similar results in an artful practice of a medical science that was continually evolving before me. It didn't take long to shatter this assumption in my clinical work with self-regulation.

Ill persons have a "limbic-visceral" sense of their illness.

I define this limbic-visceral sense as an individual's clear perception of the inner hurt associated with his illness. All sick persons experience this but few can adequately describe it to their physicians. The reason for this is simple: For the patient, the limbic-visceral sense neither involves the known (to him) anatomy nor the established tenets of known (to his physician) pathology.

VIOLATING THE LIMBIC-VISCERAL

I believe the most common mistakes we physicians make is that we violate our patients' limbic-visceral sense of their illnesses. We are trained to be—and, in most instances, are—highly focused on categorizing human suffering into one or more specific diagnostic categories. The very notion that an ill person can have a sense of his illness that is beyond our known sciences in medicine is utterly foreign to us. We find patient's accounts of their illness distracting and wasteful—and utterly irrelevant to our reimbursement codes. So it is that patients' insistence on communicating to us their innate sense of their suffering only hardens our position against them.

Until I began my clinical work with integrative medicine, I did not believe that patients' limbic-visceral senses had any relevance to my clinical work. Hence, I scrupulously resisted all their efforts to influence my *scientific* assessment of their cases by their accounts of their illness. It amazes me to look back at the first two decades of my clinical work when I failed to see the obvious fallacy of my thinking. Indeed, in spite of my best efforts, I still catch myself making three types of mistakes:

First,

> violating a patient's limbic-visceral sense of his illness;

Second,

> clinging to my belief that I am a better judge of what is and isn't pertinent in my patient's description of his suffering.

Third,

> disregarding a patient's intuitive sense of what might facilitate his healing process.

In this book and in others, I write about my unending amazement at the healing responses in injured tissues. I continue to be surprised at how chronically ill patients with ecologic, immune, nutritional and stress-related illnesses make astounding recoveries when they are able to do the right things and avoid the wrong things for a sufficiently long period of time. *The key element here is, of course, slow and steady progress.* But I didn't reach this rather sweeping conclusion without many missteps. Below I narrate brief accounts of a few of my failures with teaching autoregulation.

DISSOLVING HEADACHE

For patients with a history of chronic headache, it is my practice to carefully review information about their eating habits, food sensitivities, mold allergy, sleep and anger before I speak to the patient about my plan of management. Only after I have addressed those issues do I broach the subject of the limbic-spiritual in the management of chronic headache. Patients understand and relate to this approach well. During autoregulation classes, I outline the principles and practice of the form of self-regulation that evolved in my mind over years.

In the chapter entitled Mr. Jefferson's Headache, I describe how I learned to dissolve my migraine headache attacks with autoregulation. Each time I succeeded in controlling my headache without Demerol injections, I became excited about the potential of this approach for my patients who suffered chronic headache. In those early years, in my enthusiasm I sometimes jumped to conclusions, made some mistakes and learned some important lessens.

A man in his sixties consulted me for chronic headache. After reviewing his case history and before doing a physical examination and drawing blood for allergy tests, I made the mistake of bringing up the subject of autoregulation, and spoke enthusiastically about its value in controlling headache. Then I used the phrase "the miracle of dissolving headache." He suddenly leaned forward in his chair at the word dissolving, stared at me with searching eyes, then slumped back in his chair. I sensed his discomfort and realized that to him the word dissolving connoted some metaphysical concept. My words seem to imply to him some exotic eastern animistic ritual. Or, perhaps some sort of despicable exorcism. I tried to make a fast turnabout and talk about demonstrable, reproducible, scientific electrophysiologic parameters I use in my autoregulation laboratory to evaluate the results. He listened to me impassively, but my explanations seemed to make no impact on him.

I never saw him again.

LOOSENING UP THE BOWEL

Once Talat and I were driving back from Newport, Rhode Island. I had suffered from an intestinal virus the day before that caused nausea and intermittent abdominal cramps. Approaching New York City, we were caught in a traffic jam. My abdominal cramps gained in intensity and I needed to find a rest room. There was no exit to be seen. My discomfort grew and I became anxious.

Bowel cramps in viral infections are caused by spasm of the bowel, I reasoned. What would happen if I could loosen up the muscle in my bowel wall with autoregulation? I wondered. Wouldn't that ease off the cramps? There was nothing to lose in trying that approach. Indeed, there was no other choice.

I had heard about ancient methods that required breathing through the tissues in different body organs. Could I learn to breathe into my bowel on short notice? I wondered. If I were ever to experiment, this seemed to be the right time. In directed pulses, I could feel the energy in different parts of my body. Now I tried to feel the energy in my bowel by 'breathing' into the abdomen. To my pleasant surprise, my abdominal cramps eased off within a few breaths, and my discomfort was completely gone within a few minutes. I was excited by this new insight into autoregulation.

Some weeks after our trip to Newport, a woman professor in her fifties consulted me for ulcerative colitis. The diagnosis had been established with a biopsy. I listened to her complaints of persistent abdominal cramps, bloating and diarrhea, and thought about the prospect of teaching her how she could control some of her abdominal symptoms by loosening up the bowel with the method I found effective for myself. In my description of the method, I made the mistake of using the expression of "the miracle of clearing colon cramps" with limbic breathing. She looked at me suspiciously, recovered and smiled, but remained cold to my suggestions. I learned later that she refused the food and mold allergy tests that I had ordered.

I didn't see her again.

Later, when I realized that my approach had turned her off, I couldn't understand why an intelligent woman, a college professor, would misunderstand my intentions on such a simple issue. After all, everyone knows stress exaggerates the symptoms of ulcerative colitis. Looking back now, I can see why she might have been offended at my suggestion. I had failed to emphasize the value of my management of her food sensitivities and mold allergy in my total plan of therapies. She probably misconstrued my comments and thought that I was dismissing her colitis as an all-in-the-head problem. I would be offended too if I suffered from a disabling disorder such as ulcerative colitis and someone dismissed me as a malingerer.

LIFTING DEPRESSION
BY LIGHTING UP THE NEURONE CANDLES

To explain the nature of depression to my patients, I often use an analogy of a field of candles. All the candles in the field are wired to each other below the surface. Winds blow and extinguish some candles. When that happens, the lighted candles surrounding those that were blown out light up the extinguished candles via their below-the-surface wire connections. This is how neurotransmitter connections work at the neuronal synapses (nerve junctions) in the human brain. All neurones do not fire at all times. Some of them lose their electromagnetic potentials and become 'silent'—or extinguished in our analogy. The silent neurones are then brought back to life—are fired back up—by other neurones that surround them.

It is different in people who suffer depression. Their neurones (brain cells) crave for neurotransmitters, both of the adrenergic day and serotonergic night types. But those neurotransmitters are in short supply. Their neuronal connections—synaptic networks, in technical jargon, are weak, sometimes moribund. When the winds of sad or angry thoughts blow, they extinguish many of their neurones. The alive neurones in the vicinity of moribund neurones watch helplessly. Their links with the silent, suffering neurones are cut off. They are in no position to transfuse the moribund cells with some of their life force. Then, yet more winds of dark neurochemistry follow, putting out yet more neurones. And this goes on and on until there are no more lighted candles. There is only darkness of deepening depression—only a free fall.

One of my patients, a priest who had consulted me for chronic fatigue, asked me to see his son, back from college for Thanksgiving. The young man complained of anxiety and fatigue, and appeared depressed. He had been prescribed an antidepressant by the staff at his college campus, but had declined the prescription. The three of us talked for a while. The father had obtained good results with our program. He had become good at autoregulation and had earlier described his positive experience with this approach. I proceeded to explain to his son the basic principles and practice of autoregulation. He listened carefully. Before they left, I prescribed some nutrients for the young man.

His father returned after about two months for a follow-up visit for himself. I asked him how his son was doing at school. His face stiffened a bit. He hesitated for a while, then spoke,

> *"Dr. Ali, you missed it completely. My son was desperate for help when he saw you. Mere limbic breathing wasn't going to help him then, and it didn't. He became very depressed, suicidal. We had to see a psychiatrist who prescribed a heavy dose of Prozac to control that serious situation."*

I listened to him and admitted that I had grossly misjudged the severity of his son's condition. In my enthusiasm for autoregulation, I had completely failed to recognize that progress with autoregulation in depression can be extremely slow. Indeed, many seriously depressed individuals make no progress with autoregulation—even when combined with nutrient and herbal therapies as well as slow, sustained exercise—until their depression is lifted somewhat with antidepressants. I expressed my regrets to him, thanked him for letting me know of my error in judgment, and learned a valuable lessen.

AUTOREGULATION TAPES FOR ASTHMA

In the management of asthma, I consider immunotherapy for mold and other allergies essential to success. It is my practice to postpone such therapy until a few weeks after stabilizing the asthma situation with oral and injectable nutrient and herbal therapies, and with autoregulation.

A thoracic surgeon, and a good friend, complained of progressive wheezing and fatigue. The symptoms progressed to a degree that he was unable to keep his operating room schedule. I ordered blood tests for allergy analysis. When I saw him in my office a few days later, he smiled and said the wheezing problem was under control. He told me he was late for his own office schedule. I made the cardinal mistake of not following my usual procedures of taking a complete history and examination. In my eagerness to help him, I prescribed some nutrient therapies, gave him my autoreg tapes and asked the nurse to give him his first immunotherapy injection.

The next morning, I had a call from his wife. My friend was in hospital with an acute asthma attack. (This was one of two times that I had to face such a complication of immunotherapy in an asthmatic patient. I learned my lesson. Now, I insist on deferring mold and pollen desensitization injections for asthma patients for some weeks and use that time to teach autoregulation, and administer nutritional and herbal therapies before beginning immunotherapy.

Now that I look back, I am amazed at my naivete. How could I assume that wheezing in a thoracic surgeon can be managed any differently than in others? How could I assume that I can waive many of our treatment protocols just because the patient happens to be an experienced surgeon? How could I ever think that a thoracic surgeon can learn to control wheezing with autoregulation without diligent training in its methods?

A physician cannot make any assumptions. I had learned that as a medical student in Pakistan. I learned that again as a young surgeon in England. And I learned that again as a young pathologist in the United States. Caring for a surgeon-friend, I had to relearn the same basic rule as a not-so-young physician practicing energetic-molecular medicine.

Physicians, when seen as patients, should be seen as patients, and not as professional colleagues. Autoregulation is not an intellectual function that anyone can perfect from theory or tapes. It requires diligent work. Indeed, it is often harder for physicians to learn because of their indoctrination against self-regulation.

AM I GOING TO GET A PENICILLIN SHOT OR NOT?

A young man came to me for a recurrent sore throat. He had received multiple antibiotic injections from his other physicians. I examined him and observed that his throat was inflamed but there was no sign of pus. I talked about the dangers of excessive use of antibiotics, then spoke about some preventive measures. Next, I suggested mold and pollen allergy tests to diagnose the underlying immune problem that rendered him vulnerable to recurrent sore throat. He listened to me for a while, then asked for a penicillin injection. I repeated that a penicillin injection wasn't the answer. Furthermore, each time he took antibiotics, his general resistance would further go down. To make my points strongly, I emphasized the importance of an integrated approach with a clear focus on issues of stress and self-regulation. He interrupted me with a shrug and curtly asked, "Am I going to get a penicillin shot or not?".

His demeanor made it obvious that he considered my perspectives on the issue of health and disease as a sales pitch. Frustrated with myself for misreading the situation and bringing the issue of stress prematurely, I tried to suggest some nutrient and herbal therapies. He told me he considered his visit with me futile. I expressed my regrets and waived my office visit fee. Needless to say, I never saw him again.

Clearly, there is a right time for everything. A physician needs to develop a sense of timing, no matter how ernest he might be in his care.

****

My mistakes in clinical autoregulation which I include in this chapter, and many others that I do not, occurred during the early years of my work in energetic-molecular medicine. Now, it is extremely rare for me to make such mistakes, perhaps because I have learned to heed some useful clinical clues. Or, perhaps because most of my current patients either have read my books or have listened to my tapes before I see them. They come accepting the contribution of methods of autoregulation in the total management plan for their care.

The reward for reaching out to someone in need is not what one receives for it but what one becomes by it.

What Do Lions Know About Stress?

Chapter 9

THE BITE OF THE GRAY DOG

"Why does autoreg sometimes make the symptoms worse?" I asked Choua one day.

"Give me an example," he replied.

"My headache becomes worse when I begin autoreg," I explained.

"Autoreg makes your headache worse?" he looked puzzled. "Then why do you do it?"

"After a while the headache clears up! That's why!"

"Does that happen every time?" he asked, his curiosity piqued.

"Almost every time," I replied.

"Interesting!" Choua's eyes narrowed. "Do other people also suffer headaches when they begin autoreg?"

"No, of course not," I laughed. "Autoreg doesn't *cause* headaches. It only accentuates the perception of a headache that is already there."

"What happens to other people?"

"Their symptoms get worse," I clarified. "Sometimes, they develop new symptoms."

"New symptoms?" he frowned. "If autoreg causes new symptoms, why do they do autoreg? Some sort of self-flagellation! Is that it?"

"No, Choua. It isn't about self-flagellation. They do autoreg for the same reason I do," I replied. "After initial negative responses, their symptoms clear up just as my headache dissolves."

"Give me some examples." He became earnest. "What kind of symptoms do other people experience?"

"My patients describe three different outcomes of autoreg," I elaborated. "First, the tissues respond in a positive, comforting way. Second, the tissues..."

"You teach *other* people's tissues to respond to *you*?" he interrupted me, his eyes widening.

"No, silly, that's not the way it works," I teased.

"So, what is it that you do?" he grimaced.

"I can only help my patients perceive the energy that Nature put in their tissues."

"Uh!" Choua lightened up. "I get it now! You teach them how to attend to their bodies and perceive the tissue energy. Tell me, what is the second type of response?"

"In the second type, the tissues respond in a negative way. The response varies from brief periods of mild discomfort to severe reactions of intense distress," I continued.

"Fascinating stuff!" He cocked his head. "It's getting more interesting by the minute. Go on. And the third type of response?"

"The third outcome isn't really a response. Rather, it is an absence of response," I completed a brief description.

"Absence of response?" he frowned again, then asked, "Do you mean nothing happens?"

"Right."

"Why not?"

"That's not an easy question to answer. Maybe it is because most people go through life without ever perceiving any energy in their tissues. Indeed, most people are not aware of how human tissues can—and do—respond when one learns to attend to his tissues. Energy is an elementary aspect of living beings, and yet most persons never perceive such energy—never sense this most fundamental of all phenomena in biology. So it doesn't surprise me that much when people sense no tissue response in the beginning and simply give up."

"Your colleagues do not engage in such work, do they?"

"No. It's not taught in medical schools. Rather, it is dismissed as a taboo subject."

"Pity! It should be taught. Shouldn't it?" he asked.

"Yeah, it should be. Unfortunately, it is considered fringe medicine—fodder for the feeble-minded in medicine."

"Self-regulation for most physicians is a distraction, isn't it?" he asked sympathetically.

"Yes, it is," I confessed. "It is poorly tolerated because it interferes with surgical schedules and robs us of the great promise of miraculous drug cures."

"Tell me about the first kind of response. What kind of positive responses do your patients describe? This stuff is interesting."

"Initially, the positive responses are simple. Most people describe them as warmth or heaviness in their hands. Some talk about a sense of magnetic energy in their hands and other tissues. Yet others sense waves of energy."

"Subjective stuff, isn't it?" he asked with a smile. "Isn't that what some would dismiss as hypnotic responses to hypnotic suggestions?"

"I'm telling you what my patients tell me," I replied.

"Go on," he prodded.

"When an individual does succeed in perceiving tissue energy, it always brings profound insights into the energy dynamics in life—opens new windows, so to speak, about the visceral workings of the human body."

"It would be nice if one could put all this in a scientific mode, wouldn't it?" he asked.

"Perceptions and understanding of such tissue responses were an integral part of many tribal rituals in earlier times," I added. "The ancients understood this phenomenon well. Today, professionals in the biofeedback community accept this as a routine experience for those who practice self-regulation."

"Oh, biofeedback! Is that what you're talking about?" Choua raised his eyebrows.

"No, I'm not talking about biofeedback," I corrected him. "But certainly one can use biofeedback technology to answer your question. Every Wednesday at my autoreg lab, my patients feel energy responses and I demonstrate to them the clear electrophysiological basis of such responses. There is no mystery about it. Once you sense it, there is no..."

"Tell me, how do people describe such responses?" Choua interrupted me.

"The energy response is expressed as warmth, flushing, heaviness, tingling, throbbing, pulsation or simply as a strong magnetic sense."

"Wow!" he exclaimed. "All that really happens? Not mere illusions?"

"Many patients also express doubts about this in the beginning. But they feel reassured as they observe the changes in the energy patterns of their hearts, arteries, skin and muscles. No one can lie to himself. When the changes are there, they are real. When they are not there, that is equally real. It's that simple."

"I have no reason to doubt that," he smiled. "Let's move on to the second outcome: the negative energy responses."

"The negative energy response to self-regulation is the big question mark for me. I was hoping you might throw some light on that subject," I answered.

"Tell me, how do your patients describe the negative energy responses to autoreg?"

"The negative responses my patients describe are just as varied as the positive ones. Many people experience brief episodes of lightheadedness, anxiety, accelerated heart rate, discomfort in their eyes—with or without watering or searing effects—uneasiness in the chest, mild cramps in the abdomen, spasms in neck muscles and stiffness in lower back muscles."

"How long do such responses usually last?"

"In most instances, such responses are of short duration, lasting for a few minutes. They are of no consequence. Usually such responses are mild expressions of symptoms they have suffered in the past. Time and again, I have observed this phenomenon of pain and suffering arising from simple attempts to still the mind and perceive one's own tissue energy."

"Fascinating stuff!" Choua chugged along. "Truly fascinating stuff. What causes such responses?"

"I was hoping you might have some thoughts on the subject."

"How do I know?" he shrugged.

"Listening to body tissues is being kind to them—at least that's what everyone tells me. So why do tissues in distress protest when we try to attend to them?"

"Tissues bite back! Is that it?" he asked.

"Yeah! Sort of!" I liked the way Choua put it. "But why does that happen? What could be the energetic-molecular basis of this phenomenon?"

"They bite back," he murmured, then repeated, "Injured tissues bite back. Some sort of protest. Some rebellion. But why?"

"Yes, why?"

Choua didn't answer my question. Instead he walked over to the window and looked out. He is usually quite glib in his answers. On the few occasions when he can't come up with quick, sharp replies, he becomes a trifle testy and fidgets around. Minutes pass. If there is still no answer, he simply withdraws from the conversation. Sometimes he walks to the window and gazes at the sky, as he did that day. At other times, he simply stares at whatever object his eyes happen to fall upon. It can be a piece of paper on the floor or a door knob. Then I know I have lost him. Almost always he returns to that subject several minutes later, sometimes days or weeks later.

"The negative tissue energy responses—bites of the injured tissues, as you call them—have preoccupied me for quite some time," I began after a while, then waited for Choua's response. There was none. "Why do tissues respond to autoreg positively sometimes and negatively at others? And when tissues do not respond at all, why do they fail to do so?" I threw a volley of questions at him.

Choua obviously wasn't listening. He stood motionless at the window, making no attempt to acknowledge my questions. Then he turned and walked out.

THE BITE OF THE NECK MUSCLES

On Wednesday evenings, I conduct a three-hour autoregulation training session. As I wrote earlier, I use electrode sensors to record changing patterns of energy in the heart, blood vessels, muscles and skin. After connecting one of my patients to the computerized equipment, I lead the group through various autoreg training methods. Assuming a comfortable posture on chairs—with hands resting on thighs and palms facing upward—we close our eyes to begin meditation and energy work.

After individual periods of autoregulation lasting 10 to 15 minutes, I ask my patients to open their eyes. Next, I demonstrate the changes in the energy patterns of various body organs with moving graphs on a computer screen. In almost every session, I can point out dramatic energy changes in the different body organs of one or more patients. Almost all patients experience some tissue energy responses. With lights dimmed in the autoregulation lab, the colorful computer screen illustrates the changing patterns of the heart, muscles, blood vessels and skin. The combination of objective changes on the computer screen and perceptions of tissue energy within them is very effective in teaching my patients the principles and practice of autoregulation.

On the Wednesday following my conversation with Choua about negative energy responses, I saw him tiptoe into the autoreg lab as I led the group into energy work. He took a seat in the back and looked around to see what others in the room were doing. He assumed the same posture as everyone else, closed his eyes and began to follow my lead. I suppressed a smile, closed my eyes and continued my work.

The first person I wired for autoreg that evening was Sheila, a 48-year-old woman who consulted me for sinusitis, chronic headache and fatigue.

She had received some biofeedback training previously and was skeptical about any other form of self-regulation. Nonetheless, she attended my autoregulation workshop, she returned for autoregulation training in our laboratory. I applied the electrodes and other sensors for monitoring various body functions. Then I asked her to sit comfortably on her chair, close her eyes and listen.

During the first few minutes of autoregulation training, I usually observe the subjects and their moving graphs on the computer screen. I note how cortical or limbic their state of biology is. (Sharp fluctuations in graph lines with tall peaks and deep valleys indicate stressful cortical turbulence, and smooth even lines with gentle waves reflect a healing limbic calmness). Sheila's neck visibly stiffened as she closed her eyes, and the computer screen displayed wild fluctuations in her graphs of skin conductance energy, muscle potentials, heart rate and pulse pressure. Quite common, this response merely indicates apprehension at not knowing what will follow. Generally, such electromagnetic fluctuations subside and I begin to see objective

---

evidence of a transition from a stressful, turbulent cortical state to an even, restorative limbic profile, but this was not to be the case with Sheila.

Within several moments, Sheila's neck began to turn and twist. She frowned with closed eyes. Her lips quivered, and her jaw muscles tensed. A few moments later, she broke into clonic, almost convulsive spasms of her twisted neck. To witness sudden, unexpected convulsive activity in a patient who appeared in good health is not unusual experience for physicians. I had seen such events in emergency department many times. I am rarely unnerved in such clinical situations. But, I found Sheila's twisted neck and her distorted facial features frightening. I suppose it happened because it was so utterly unexpected. I touched Sheila's hand and asked her to open her eyes. Her clonic neck contractions stopped as suddenly as they appeared once she'd opened her eyes.

I forced a smile and made some general comments. A faint smile appeared on Sheila's face. We were quiet for a few moments.

"What was that?" I asked, in as natural a tone as I could muster.

"Oh, it's nothing," Sheila replied evenly.

"Nothing?" I asked, surprised at her composure.

"It's nothing. It happens all the time."

"Happens all the time?"

"Yes! I am used to it."

"What is it? How often do you get it? I mean, why didn't you tell me about it?"

"Happens all the time." Sheila forced another smile. "I didn't tell you because I thought there was no point to it."

"No point to it?" I was incredulous.

"No other doctor believed me. So I didn't see any point in bothering you with it. I guess the doctors thought it was hysteria or something."

"Maybe it is. Maybe it isn't. Why don't you tell me about it?" I coaxed her.

"Oh! Dr. Ali, there is nothing anyone can do about it. You know, it happens every night." Sheila's voice quivered. "Every night, it happens."

I looked at her in silence for a few moments. She looked back at me impassively.

"Tell me more about it." I broke the silence.

"There is nothing more to tell." She shrugged.

"What happens afterward?"

"Every night it happens as I put my head on my pillow and close my eyes. My neck turns and twists and cramps. It hurts me awful." Sheila suddenly broke down and sobbed.

"Do you want to stop here?" I asked sympathetically, offering her a box of tissue paper.

"When my neck hurts, I open my eyes and the spasms go away," she continued a moment later. "Sometimes I sit up and think. Sometimes I try to read. Then I get exhausted and try again, and again it happens. This goes on all night. Every night."

"When do you sleep?"

"When I am totally exhausted with pain and sleeplessness. Sometimes in the early hours of the morning, maybe four or five, I finally doze off for a few minutes," Sheila sobbed again.

I sat frozen as I listened to her. Tolstoy thought happy people were all alike, but each unhappy person was unhappy in his own way. How many Sheilas did he listen to? I wondered. How many Sheilas are there in this world anyway? Living out their lives in silos of sadness.

"Sheila, would you do me a favor?" I asked her, recovering from my personal thoughts. "Would you mind if we did this again?"

"What would that do?" she asked indifferently.

"We might learn something," I encouraged her.

"Learn something?" Sheila smiled again. "Go ahead, if you think it will help *you*."

Her sarcasm didn't escape me. I hesitated for a minute. Now that I write about Sheila I wonder if I knew why I made this request. I knew it was going to distress her again. What did I hope to find? Scientific curiosity taking wing at someone else's expense. Did I know what might happen next? If I did, how did I? It's odd that these questions never arose until now that I write about it, a few years after that event.

"Yes Sheila, I think it will help me," I admitted.

"Let's do it then." Sheila shrugged.

"Can you take the pain if I continue for a few minutes this time?" I asked.

"Take the pain?" She laughed this time. "What else do I do every night?"

"Sheila, this time I am going to close my eyes, too. We will do autoreg together."

We started again. Sheila closed her eyes and the neck contractions returned just as they had the first time. I braced myself, led her into autoregulation again and closed my own eyes. Long hours of autoregulation had given me the ability to turn off my own cortical monkey on rather short notice. I opened my eyes after what seemed to me were five to seven minutes. Sheila's neck still quivered a little, but the intense clonic contractions were gone. Her face appeared calm, her hands resting limp and loose on her thighs. I asked her to open her eyes. We talked for some minutes and then did some more autoregulation. In the end, I asked Sheila to return for some more training.

****

"Why did Sheila's muscles go into spasms when she closed her eyes?" Choua asked as he joined me in my office after the autoregulation class.

"It's almost midnight, Choua," I replied. "Time to go home. There is a tumor board meeting at the hospital early tomorrow morning and I have to present three cases of cancer."

"The cortical monkey doesn't let up, does it?" he continued.

"What does the cortical monkey have to do with Sheila's neck muscle spasms?" I asked, puzzled.

"It doesn't know how to let go," he replied evenly. "I want to tell you a story."

"I like your stories, Choua, but it's late," I said politely, "and your stories tend to be long. How about tomorrow morning."

"During the tumor board meeting," Choua chuckled. "Not a bad time to tell stories."

"No, I didn't mean that," I added hastily. Choua often distracts me with his stories during the long meetings at the hospital, which I am required to attend. "Not during the tumor board meeting. I am presenting three cases with complex cancer-related problems. Maybe after it."

"Maybe," he smiled and watched me stuff my papers into

my briefcase. Then we walked out to the parking lot together.

Next morning, Choua joined me in the tumor board meeting. He took the seat next to me. As the oncologist discussing the cases approached the podium, Choua leaned and asked, "Why did Sheila's neck muscles rebel when she closed her eyes?"

"I need to listen closely to the presenter, Choua," I whispered in his ear, "because I have to respond to specific questions he raises about the case when it is my turn to discuss the biopsy and surgical specimen."

"An interesting question, isn't it?" he continued, undeterred. "Why did the neck contractions stop when she opened her eyes?"

"I don't know!" I whispered, harshly this time.

"And why did the neck muscles finally respond when Sheila and you persevered?" Choua pressed.

"Oh shush, Choua, for God's sake," I elbowed him angrily.

"Why do injured tissues bite back?" he muttered as he pulled away from me.

"We'll talk after this conference is over," I tried a conciliatory approach, recognizing that confrontation wasn't working.

"Fine! Fine!" He leaned toward me again. "I didn't mean to distract you."

"So gracious of you, Choua," I replied sarcastically.

The purpose of autoregulation, of course, is to comfort the hurt tissues, my thoughts began to wander. Why did Sheila's tissues bite back? I rubbed my face and tried to listen to the oncologist. What possible good did her neck muscles think could come from the games they played? Was it anger turned in, as my friends in psychiatry propose? Was it spite? Sheer hostility of the tissues? Did these tissues act so viciously on their own or did they take their cues from somewhere else? I thought about many other Sheilas who had described negative responses of different kinds. The main theme was always the same. But why? Why do tissues respond in a comforting, healing way one time and in a hurting way at others? Choua glibly talked about the injured tissues biting back. But why?

I do not recall how long I remained lost in my reverie. The next thing I remember is Choua elbowing me to draw my attention. Everyone in the room was staring at me. The conference moderator had obviously called upon me and I seemed to be the only person in the room not to know that. I gave a flustered look to Choua, picked up my papers and awkwardly walked to the podium. It was obvious to everyone in the conference room that I had not been paying any attention to the moderator. There was no point in trying to trick anyone into thinking otherwise. Silence, at such times, is merciful.

I left the conference room briskly after presenting my material, not wanting to linger among my colleagues after the fiasco caused by Choua. I sensed he was following me and moved faster.

"Sheila's energy dynamics got very confused," Choua spoke in a soft tone as he finally caught up with me.
"There is a time for everything," I complained bitterly.
"I'm sorry," he looked at me the way I have seen Sidney, our son Omar's pug, look at him after he has had an accident.
"You're too much, Choua," I said, softening. "Confused? Why did Sheila's neck muscles get confused?"
"They just did."
"Not angry?" I asked, forgetting my fury. "Not hostile? Just plain confused? Why?"
"Yes," he replied evenly. "Simply and plainly confused."

We walked in silence for several moments. Choua has the capacity to engage in more than one conversation at a time—in one, he listens to another person but doesn't respond, and in the other, he conducts an internal dialogue that people in his company know nothing about. I had a sense Choua spoke to himself more than he did to me on our way back to the laboratory. Back at my office, he picked up a journal on my desk and buried his face in it.

DO MOLECULES, CELLS AND TISSUES HAVE CONSCIOUSNESS?

"Do tissues have consciousness?" Choua asked after several minutes.

"I have been told that what separates man from beast is consciousness," I replied. "Man, as conventional wisdom holds, is capable of rational thought. Hence, he is rational."

"Where do human tissues fit in this scheme of things?" he groused. "With man, the rational being, or with the beast, the living thing without any consciousness?"

"Human tissues are globs of protoplasm. Do they have any consciousness? I don't know," I replied.

"Ugly clumps of cells, blood and tissue fluid! Is that it?"

"What's your point, Choua?" I asked.

"So what are human tissues?" he ignored my question. "Heaps of living matter? Is that all there is to human tissues?"

"You know about such things. I don't."

"Sheila's neck muscles. Why did they go into spasms? Confused tissues, ever so ready to rebel and become spastic? They cannot be trusted anytime, anywhere? Poor thing! She closed her eyes for a few moments and the confused muscles strike. Without the constant censor of her thinking head, Sheila's neck muscles go crazy, and quiver with rage!"

"Is this conversation taking us any place?" I asked in frustration. "Do human tissues have consciousness or not?"

"I do not know much about the consciousness," Choua continued. "So, I don't know whether tissues and molecules do or do not have consciousness. The gurus of artificial intelligence talk about computer models of consciousness. They claim that the "problem of consciousness" is on the verge of solution. I don't understand such matters, but I do know this: The injured tissues do not lie. The only part of the human condition that lies to us is the thinking brain. The heart, the lungs, the kidneys, muscles, tendons and the skin never learned to lie. When we do choose to listen to the injured tissues, they speak the truth. If the tissues are in pain, they say so. This is the truth about the language of injured tissues. This is the truth about the bite of injured tissues."

"How do you know?" I challenged Choua.

"Because I know that tissues are not into biting," he posited. "Living tissues are loving beings. When they bite, they do so out of pain and confusion—and not to spite anyone. Nor do they do so out of anger. Sheila will find that out with time."

Choua looked at me intently for a while, then laughed lightly and walked out.

****

Several months later, Sheila told me how autoreg had cleared most of her neck muscle spasms, except for some nights when she had been extremely stressed during the day.

The Gray Dog

Some days later, Choua told me this story:

A boy brought home two newborn puppies, one was white and the other gray. He fell in love with the white puppy. He put the gray puppy in a crib and held the white puppy in his hands. The white puppy kept his eyes closed. His skin was soft and his hair snow-white and delicate. The boy petted his white puppy until late evening hours. Then he asked his mother if he could put his puppy to sleep in his own bed. His mother smiled and told him that was very dangerous. The puppy could be smothered by him in his sleep. The boy understood that and gently put the puppy in his crib.

When he woke up the next morning, his puppies were awake and seemed hungry. He took the puppies out of their crib and asked his mother to teach him how to prepare their formula. As he fed them, he had eyes only for the white puppy. Then he put the puppies back into the crib, instructed his mother about their care and left for school. At school, he was distracted all day by thoughts of his white puppy. The gray puppy was not a part of his day. When the school bell rang for the last time, he ran home to be with his white puppy. Once home, he threw his satchel on a chair and rushed to the crib. The noise woke up the puppies. He lifted both puppies out of the crib and put them on the floor. Again, he had eyes only for the white puppy. He petted him and held him in his lap. The gray puppy moved around, unaware and unaffected by the boy's preoccupation with the white puppy. Late that night, he fed the puppies again, his eyes remaining fixed on the white puppy.

The next day was no different. The boy woke up and hurried to the crib. The puppies were sleeping. He gently petted the white puppy as it slept. Then he brought the puppies their meal. He watched every little movement the white puppy made. The day at school was like the one before. He thought about his tiny white puppy. Again, the gray puppy was out of his mind. That afternoon and evening, he again played with the white puppy. The gray puppy wandered around, oblivious to the boy's preoccupation with the white puppy.

Days passed and then weeks. The boy's fondness for the white puppy seemed to grow with each passing day. The puppies grew up fast and became strong. The boy started housebreaking his puppies. That's when the boy's parents noticed that the gray puppy began to misbehave. Sometimes he looked at the boy with silent, plaintive eyes, at other times he barked without any reason. On occasion, he appeared to want to break things. On some afternoons, the gray puppy seemed to purposely throw up his food on the kitchen floor and soil the rug in the living room. That annoyed the boy's parents and they scolded him. As for the boy, he was too absorbed playing with his white puppy to want to do much with the gray puppy. Each time the gray puppy did something the boy didn't like, it drove the boy even closer to his white puppy. The more the gray puppy was scolded, the more accident prone he became.

Months passed. The puppies grew up into little dogs. The boy's love for his white dog grew deeper with each passing month. The white dog knew this. He waited for the boy to return from school all day. The afternoons were pure bliss for both of them.

They played together, ate their meals together and then went out to a nearby field for more play. The gray dog seemed to sense the closeness between the two and often became sad. Sometimes he felt angry and hurt. On most days, he kept all that to himself, but sometimes it was too much for him. That was when the accidents would happen, the ones that made the boy angry. Some more months passed.

Then the gray dog changed. He was not sad anymore. Nor was he ever angry. No one noticed that the gray dog stopped having accidents. He neither made a mess in the kitchen nor soiled the rugs anymore. When the boy returned home, the gray dog stood back, watching the white dog leap to meet his little master. Sometimes when the boy's eyes fell upon the gray dog, the dog gently cocked his head or wagged his tail. That was all. The boy didn't follow it with any words. The gray dog didn't ask for anything more.

Years passed. The boy grew up into a young man and the dogs into two strong dogs. Every day, when the young man returned from work, the white dog greeted him with great excitement and leaped all over him. The gray dog stood behind, silently watching the two friends. After some time, the man went to his kitchen and cooked his meal as the white dog hovered around him. The gray dog stood still in the corner, his eyes blank and unexpressive. After the meal was ready, the man ate it with his white dog and then left his house for a walk with his white dog. It was then that the gray dog walked over to the table and ate the leftovers. Then he walked out briskly to catch up with the man and his white dog. There he stood by the edge of the field, impassively looking at the man and the white dog. When it turned dark, the man and his white dog returned home; the gray dog walking several paces behind them. That was the way weeks followed days and months followed weeks.

One rainy day the man was driving to work when his car slid and crashed into another car. He sustained a head injury and concussion and fractured several ribs. Some days later, he opened his eyes and saw some fuzzy figures in white robes milling around his bed. He tried to sit up but collapsed with pangs of pain in different parts of his body. Moments later, he opened his eyes and looked around the room. He saw tubes and wires running into his body parts from bottles hanging from poles and video screens on the walls. Is it a nightmare? Am I dying? he wondered. Then he saw some nurses walk by. He realized he was in a hospital. He thought back and recalled the fleeting moment of terror before his car crashed. His body shook with fear. He tried to get up, felt a sharp pain in his chest and collapsed onto his bed. Am I going to live? he asked himself as he came around the second time. He looked out the window. The sunset filtered weakly through the mist of a late winter afternoon.

The man closed his eyes. A faint shadow of a dog appeared in the distant mist. Then the shadow sharpened into the face of a white dog. The dog looked at him with gleaming eyes. My dog, he murmured softly and opened his eyes. His face softened into a smile. A nurse passed by. Again he closed his eyes to recapture the image of his white dog and savor the moment. The dog's head reappeared. His chest heaved as he looked longingly at his dog. Love filled his whole body and everything that surrounded him. He opened his eyes and looked around. He felt calm as he looked at the pale yellow solution dripping slowly into the little chamber below the IV bottle and the blips and waves moving across the heart monitor.

The man studied the ICU room for a while and then closed

his eyes again, wondering if his white-faced visitor still hung around in the mist outside his window. As his eyes closed, the image of his white dog reappeared, and then it changed. The white face of the dog became pale and then beige. Slowly the color deepened and turned darker. Suddenly, there stood before him his gray dog, silent and sullen and sad. Something stirred in him. He opened his eyes in pain. The image of the head of his gray dog vanished. He looked at the faint pale sun disk through the mist and felt sadness surging within him. Slowly he closed his eyes. A sharp image hit his eyes this time. It was the picture of his puppies the day he first brought them home. Something stirred in him again, much more intensely than before. He opened his eyes but this time it was different. The image of the gray dog persisted in the mist. The gray dog peered at him with his large, soft brown eyes. Oh, my God! The words froze in his throat. How could I? How could anyone? He cried out in pain. How could anyone be so cruel? How could I have been so cruel, and for so long? He closed his eyes in deep anguish. The image of the gray dog persisted. The dog looked at him with vacant eyes. The man's arms rose to reach the gray dog in the mist. The dog's image receded further back into the mist. And then the dog's eyes turned wet and there was a flood of tears in his large, brown eyes. Oh, my God! The man winced with intense pain. How could I? How could anyone? How could I? He repeated his words. But the images rolled on and on, like a homemade video. Images of a tiny gray puppy, searching for something in the eyes of a little boy. Images of a gray puppy awkwardly throwing himself at a little boy as the boy shrank back to pick up a white puppy. Images of a puppy vomiting on a kitchen floor and urinating on a rug. Images of a puppy being scolded by his parents. Images of a gray dog barking and breaking things and being punished. Images of a dog standing still in the corner sadly looking at a white dog and his master eating their meal on a table. Oh, my God! How could I? How could anyone?

The man trembled uncontrollably as he wept unashamedly. 'God, take me if you will,' he sobbed inconsolably, 'but first let me make it up to my gray dog'.

The man survived his injuries and was let out of the hospital after some days. He took a taxi to his home. As the taxi drove onto his driveway, the dogs heard the noise and ran to the front door. The white dog was ahead of the gray dog as had been their habit for years. The man stepped out of the taxi. The white dog thrashed against the door with full force of his forelegs, in a frenzy of motion. The gray dog peered out from behind the white dog, his whole body heaving with excitement and his tail wagging wildly. The door suddenly gave, spilling the white dog. The dog lunged at his master. The gray dog leaped behind him and then came to an abrupt halt. The man gently pushed the white dog aside, threw his arms wide open, ran toward the gray dog and hugged him.

The gray dog bit the man.

WHY DID THE GRAY DOG BITE THE MAN?

"Tell me why did the gray dog bite his master?" I asked Choua when he returned a few days later. "Was he angry? Did he want to avenge himself?"

Choua turned his head to look at me, opened his mouth to say something, then picked up a journal from my desk and began to read.

"What did the gray dog want?" I continued my questions. "Revenge for all those years of neglect? Of hurt? Of absence of love?"

"How could he have known what had passed before his master's eyes in the hospital intensive care unit?" he asked, without looking up from the journal.

"Obviously the gray dog knew nothing of what had transpired in the hospital. The events in the intensive care unit couldn't have anything to do with the reason the dog bit his master."

"How could the dog have known anything about what his master felt on the day of his return from the hospital that day?" he ignored my remarks.

"Right! The dog couldn't have known any of that. So why did he bite the man?"

"How could he have known he was going to be hugged that day?" Choua went on.

"Yes! Yes!" I said, with irritation. "Why do you keep asking those rhetorical questions?"

"Had he been scheming silently for years for that day to arrive?" Choua continued with his question, his head still buried in the pages of the journal, oblivious to the irritation in my voice. "So he could bite him and get even for years of suffering? How could he have figured all that in the one brief moment when the man brushed aside his beloved white dog and ran to him?"

"Do you expect me to answer your questions?" I asked impatiently.

"Could it be that the gray dog was simply confused?" He raised his head from the journal and looked at me for the first time since he entered my office.

"The confusion thing again!" I mused. "Just like Sheila's neck spasms.

"Yeah! Just like Sheila's neck contractions," he replied.

"Why then? Why not on some earlier day?" I asked, thoroughly befuddled.

"Could the master's hug have stunned the dog? Could he suddenly have gotten disoriented by an unexpected burst of love? Love coming from someone he thought incapable of loving him?"

I wondered about Choua's explanation. Not entirely without merit. Choua was lost in his thoughts, oblivious to all my questions. Then he backed away from the window and walked out.

Why did the gray dog bite his master anyway? Was he angry? Vengeful? What did he want? Revenge for all the years of neglect, of hurt, of absence of love?

IF BAD THOUGHTS CAN CAUSE CANCER, WHY CAN'T GOOD THOUGHTS CURE IT?

"If bad thoughts can cause cancer," we heard an expert pronounce on the radio some time ago, "why can't good thoughts make it go away?" The expert then went on to congratulate himself for the clarity of his thoughts.

"Do you think this expert has ever cared for anyone with cancer?" Choua asked.

"I don't think he is a physician," I replied.

"He is right about the first part of his discovery," Choua chuckled. "Indeed, unrelenting bad thoughts can create relentless stress that can break our molecular and energy defenses, and so lead to the production of tumors. How does this expert know that the tumor cells—or for that matter healthy cells—care about our infatuation with mind-over-body healing notions?"

"Everyone seems to believe in the mind-over-body theory these days," I replied.

"Who told him that mere thoughts can metamorphose into the physical reality of one's choosing? Have any of your patients ever told you that?"

"No, at least I don't remember."

"*The injured tissues respond only when they want to, heeding internal cues.* Isn't that what you see in autoreg lab every day?"

"Yes, in a way that's true."

"What you call the 'unthinking mode'. Tissues do not care much about the great intellectual prowess of the mind-over-body gurus, do they?"

"No, I don't think they do," I confessed.

"Injured tissues have little respect for the clever intellectual schemes foisted on gullible people by new-age gurus, don't they?" Choua asked sarcastically.

I see many patients who tell me they can control their migraine headaches and asthma attacks with mind control. Someone once told me he even "killed" his cancer by turning off its blood supply. This always fascinates me. I do not for a single moment doubt that they are telling me the truth as *they* see it. So I ask them to explain how they use their minds to control their headaches or asthma attacks. This is how the conversations have gone many times: (text reproduced from *RDA: Rats, Drugs and Assumptions).*

"Tell me, how do you control your asthma attack?" I ask.

"By mind control," the patient replies.

"Good! Now, tell me how do you do mind control?" I ask again.

"By mind-over-body," the patient repeats.

"That's good. How do you do your mind-over-body thing?" I repeat.

"You know how! By mind-over-body."

"That's really wonderful. Now tell me how do you do it?"

"By ... By mind over ..."

"Yes, I know it is by mind-over-body. But tell me how you do it," I persist. "I write about this stuff. I can't write mind-over-body over and over again, can I?"

There is usually a long pause. Then comes a hesitant answer:

"I guess I really don't know. But honest, Doc, it has

happened many times," he speaks defensively.

"Of course, it has happened many times," I reassure him.

I believe him. I have no valid reason to call his assertion a lie or consider it a delusional plausibility. I do, however, have a strong sense that the asthma attack does not subside because he has figured out a way to send some clever electromagnetic impulses from his thinking cortical brain to the tightened muscles in his bronchial tubes. Rather, by some great intuitive insight he has learned to keep his thinking mind (cortical monkey, in autoregulation terminology) out of the way of his bronchial tubes. Delivered from the ceaseless chatter of the mind, the limbic muscles in the bronchial tube open up. They do so because that's what they were designed to do. The bronchial muscles do not know how to write computer software. Neither do they know how to read poetry. They open up because that's the only thing they know how to do. The thinking mind can shut them off, but it doesn't know how to open them up. That they must do by themselves, through some limbic quality, without any help from the cortical monkey.

THE BITE OF CONFUSED BRAIN CHEMISTRY

Edward ran a profitable engineering company before he was hospitalized for suicidal depression. He suffered from multiple allergies and chemical sensitivities. Prior to and after his hospitalization, Edward consulted a succession of psychiatrists who prescribed almost every single antidepressant described in the *Physician's Desk Reference*. He reacted to all of them except Klonopin, which he took but tolerated poorly. His depression fluctuated widely, and he often became suicidal. His wife, Susan, brought him to me one winter evening. She had learned of my work with nondrug therapies. Susan was hoping, she told me, that diagnosis and management of allergies and chemical sensitivities and nutrient therapies might alleviate some of his depression. All through the first visit, he remained distant and doubtful.

In those early years of my work with environmental medicine and autoregulation, I had the opportunity to care for a large number of patients with allergies and chemical sensitivities who also suffered from depression. Depression in such patients, even when there is a family history of depression, responds well to nondrug management therapies of molecular medicine. None of those patients, however, had been so afflicted with deep, unrelenting depression. I felt inadequate and unsure of my ability to manage such an advanced case. Still, I knew that optimal care of allergies and chemical sensitivities, proper nutritional support and autoregulation could be expected to relieve some of his suffering. My main task was to make sure Edward and his wife understood that. They seemed to and told me to go ahead. Uncertain of myself, I proceeded with the examination and micro-elisa allergy tests. During the next visit I reviewed the test results, initiated immunotherapy, prescribed nutrient therapies and gave him training in basic autoregulation. As Susan looked on with hope, Edward remained skeptical.

During the next follow-up visit, Edward looked distraught and annoyed. I asked him how he felt.

"You want the truth, Doc?" he asked with unmasked hostility.
"Yes!" I answered.
"I think this whole thing is a hoax," Edward said flatly.

"A hoax?" I was taken aback.

"Yes. A hoax—hoax to make money!" Edward frowned.

Edward's words caught me off guard. This was the first time anyone had accused me in this way. I looked at Susan and fumbled for words. Susan looked embarrassed. I looked out the window for a few brief moments. The sky always has a comforting quality for me.

"Shall we stop here?" I asked Edward as I recovered.

"I don't care. You do what you want to do," he answered indifferently.

I looked at Susan. She told me they had driven for more than an hour to come to Bloomfield, and asked me if I would continue. Edward simply shrugged his shoulders. Still tentative, I proceeded.

A week later, Susan told me Edward was now very intrigued by my basic concept of energy-over-mind, the energy of body tissues as the medium of self-regulation. He listened to my tapes, read and re-read *The Cortical Monkey and Healing* and some of my other writings on this subject. His initial doubts appeared to have been replaced with curiosity. He had some problems with alcohol abuse and had attended some meetings of AA and other support groups. He stopped going to those meetings because he had not found them to be very helpful.

The promise of autoregulation, Edward told Susan, was totally different. What appealed to him most was the central idea of autoregulation—of seeking healing with energy, a no-thinking rather than a clever-thinking approach. During one of the early autoregulation training sessions, he felt pulses in his fingertips and became very excited about it, but then it didn't happen again. Still, he persisted with autoregulation.

Days passed, then weeks. Pulses didn't return to his fingertips, nor did any other part of his body respond during autoregulation. Edward read the books again and listened to tapes endlessly. Nothing happened.

The patches of snow on the north side of the woods around our office in Blairstown melted away and bulbs began to sprout. Ground squirrels seemed happy in their spring celebratory dance. On many visits, Susan brought along her teenage sons. Strikingly good-looking boys, they made a handsome family, close, loving and full of life — at least that's the way they looked to people who didn't know the deep river of anguish that flowed within them. The boys understood the enormous inner pain of their father and the unending misery of their mom.

Some more weeks passed and Edward continued to suffer, often intensely. He practiced autoregulation regularly, he told me, but there had been no response from any of his tissues. After a few months of persisting, he felt some pulses in his fingertips for a few brief moments in the shower, and then, in his own words, his fingers went dead.

I could think of no clear approach. I began to consider the futility of this tack for him. Still, I advised him to persist. His allergy symptoms abated somewhat, but overall there was no appreciable improvement. Hope was fading from Susan's face. Such times are hard on physicians. Would it ever work for Edward? Am I chasing a delusion? I asked myself.

In late August that year, I conducted a weekend

autoregulation workshop for physicians in my office. It seems so improbable now, but I asked Edward if he would attend the workshop. I didn't expect him to understand the technical discussion of the energy and molecular foundation of autoregulation, but I thought he might experience a breakthrough during the extended periods of autoregulation we practiced at the workshop. Or perhaps, at some deeper, visceral level I was seeking vindication of my therapies that were clearly unproven and could have been easily misconstrued. Edward agreed to come.

Before I began the workshop, I took Edward aside and told him to sit by the back door so he could quietly leave the room if he became uncomfortable at any time. Edward attentively listened to the introductory lectures, though he couldn't hide his frustration at not being able to understand the medical jargon. Then we all went into autoregulation and closed our eyes. Within minutes, I sensed some turmoil in the back of the room and opened my eyes to see Edward's back as he hurried out. This is what he told me later when we walked out for lunch:

"Dr. Ali, it was awful! God awful! I closed my eyes and I felt this huge, powerful hand reach down from the darkness above, sharply twist my neck and try to yank my head through the ceiling. I just had to get out. I'm sorry, Dr. Ali. I am very sorry. I know what you are trying to do. But it's no use."

FIELDS OF CANDLES

Depression is a problem of confused brain chemistry, I tried to explain to Edward when I saw him after the fiasco at the physician's meeting. I told him to imagine a field of candles. Below the surface, all candles were wired. When the winds blew, many of the candles were put out. The circuitry connecting the candles beneath the surface came to life and lit the extinguished candles. It all happened in moments. No one realized that one candle had gone out. No one, of course, who had intact circuitry.

When cells are hit hard by injurious elements, be they chemical injuries to nerve cells or sad thoughts that deplete the energy neurotransmitters at the cell membranes, the cells recover, largely because they *network*. (Cells learned to network long before ivy leaguers knew anything about it.) The candles in the cells are lit up by electromagnetic matchsticks sent to them by their friendly neighbor cells.

It is different with people who suffer from depression. Their cells crave for the day (adrenergic) and night (serotergic) neurotransmitters, but the neurotransmitters are nowhere to be found. Their network connections are weak, sometimes moribund. When the winds blow, they put out the candles. The cells in the neighborhood watch helplessly. Then there are yet more winds and yet more candles go out. And it goes on and on till, as one patient who suffers from depression and who listened to me talk about the fields of candles put it, there are no more lit candles. There is only the darkness of deep depression. Deep holes that sink deeper and deeper. And there are no walls around the holes. Only a free fall into abysmal darkness.

I told Edward I had seen people learn how to banish those winds of the thinking mind when they first feel them rising. I had seen what limbic tissue energy can do. I had seen all that through the eyes of my patients who had been there. There, deep in those dark recesses. I also wondered where true hope ended and deception began. I wondered if the experience of these other people had any relevance to Edward.

I don't know why and how Edward persisted with autoregulation. Some months later, disillusioned with the results, I suggested to Edward and Susan that they consult some other physicians who might have better luck than I did. "Doc, if you want to throw me out, do it. I am not going to see any more doctors. I have seen enough for one lifetime," Edward answered emphatically.

It took Edward several months before he began to feel his tissues respond to autoregulation. He told me he was able to do things at home and sometimes at work, and didn't much think about the relief that death might bring anymore. My notes written on Edward's chart include the following quotation from Susan, "After nineteen years, Edwards has lived this summer." I was deeply moved by her words. Edward followed it by telling me how successfully he was coping with heavy, ongoing losses at his business and how he was dealing with the possibility of declaring bankruptcy.

"Doc, it is hard to believe I am doing all this and still continue to think of the future of my family," he told me one day.

How much punishment can a person take? No one knows enough to be a pessimist, wrote Norman Cousins. I wondered what he might have meant by that. There is a limit, an absolute limit to how much anyone can suffer before total disintegration. Cousins must have known that.

What can Edward do to absorb these new shocks? I wondered. I advised him to consider joining the local Recovery chapter in his area and attend their group meetings, now that his body was beginning to respond. Edward and Susan listened to me intently.

"Doc, you're a very funny man," Edward's face broke into a broad grin.

"What did I say that's so funny?" I asked, somewhat overwhelmed by his sudden outburst of energy.

"You are funny! Doc, very funny," he went on as his wife looked at him with obvious confusion.

"Yes! I am funny, Edward. But I still don't know what you found so funny," I said.

"Doc! How could you tell me to go to Recovery group meetings?"

"Because I think folks at Recovery are very good at what they do," I answered matter-of-factly.

"Doc, you forget what I told you when I first saw you. Remember I told you I had been to AA and several church-organized support groups. I told you the talking therapies had not worked for me. You are the one who first told me to try the tissue energy approach. You are the one who first talked to me about listening to tissues. Perceiving their energy as you call it. Enhancing it. And when the tissues wouldn't talk back to me, you told me to hang on. So I hung on. Boy, did I hang on! I bought all that. And now that things are beginning to shape up, you tell me to return to those group meetings. You are funny! Doc, you're a very funny man." Edward stopped talking and looked at me like the cat that swallowed the canary.

LUPUS ON THE HEELS OF MOM'S DEATH, MULTIPLE SCLEROSIS ON THOSE OF DIVORCE

Tammy, a woman in her late forties, consulted me for multiple sclerosis. She had experienced abnormal sensations in her limbs with "pins and needles" and weakness of muscles for a few months. She became very frightened when she started losing her balance and had difficulty walking. MRI scans ordered by one neurologist showed demyelinating lesions in her brain and spinal cord. A second MRI scan ordered by a second neurologist confirmed the diagnosis of multiple sclerosis.

"I know it's not that," Tammy spoke after I finished reading her file and looked up.

"It's not what?" I asked, without really needing any clarification of her words.

"It's not multiple sclerosis," she said firmly.

"How do you know?"

"I just know."

"How?" I persisted.

"Because that's what happened the last time," she replied emphatically.

"What happened last time?"

"They said it was lupus and they gave me cortisone. I threw the cortisone out after a few weeks."

"Then what?"

"Then I took a lot of vitamins and my lupus went away."

"How was lupus diagnosed," I asked, feigning ignorance.

"They did all the tests. ANA, LE prep and a test for proteins in the urine. You know, everything the rheumatologists do."

I had gotten used to such stories by then. The first few times had been different. It had been hard to believe patients who told me such stories. It literally meant throwing out all my medical texts. Patients with serious autoimmune disorders, such as lupus and multiple sclerosis, are not supposed to get better by simply taking vitamin pills, at least not according to our medical texts. The hard-nosed pathologist in me had great difficulty believing what medical texts said couldn't be believed. Then things changed for me. My patients forced me to think differently. With the passing years, I saw many patients who were told they had lupus with positive lupus tests and go on to recover completely and live healthy lives. Similarly I saw patients with arthritis and positive rheumatoid tests who recovered. I realized the tests merely indicate stress on our immune defenses. The injured and confused immune system begins to make destructive antibodies. Positive lupus and rheumatoid tests were merely that. Nothing more. How many times does one have to be hit on his head?

"Tell me something about the stress in your life." I returned from my own thoughts.

"You know how it is. Everyone suffers stress in life," she replied.

"That's true. Still, tell me. Is he very supportive?" I asked her, gesturing to her husband who sat silently listening to us.

"Yeah, he is supportive," she replied after a slight, initial hesitation.

We physicians do learn with time. Minor delays in answers often tell us more than many carefully crafted answers from our patients. I smiled at her husband and returned to my questions.

"When did they tell you that you had lupus?" I asked.
"1984." Tammy leaned back in the chair.
"What happened in '84?"
"Nothing!"
"What happened in '83?"
"Nothing!"
"Nothing in '84 and nothing in '83?" I looked into her eyes, persisting with my inquiry.
"What happened in 83?" Tammy sat up.
"Yes, what happened in 83?"
"My mother died." Tammy's neck stiffened.
"Were you close?"
"Very."
"Very close?"
"She was my best friend."
"What happened early this year?"
"What do you mean?"
"What happened in the months before you developed pins and needles in legs and arms?"

A hurt expression crossed Tammy's face and she leaned forward in her chair. I looked at her in silence. She seemed to read my mind and quickly recovered her composure. Then she turned her face to her husband who glanced at me uncomfortably. I looked back at Tammy.

"We had family troubles."
"Would you rather not talk about them?" I asked.
"No! There's nothing to hide. We separated for some

months."

"And then?"

"Then we got together to see if we could make it."

"And then?"

"And then we realized it had to end. There had to be a divorce."

Tammy broke down. I didn't have to look at her husband to learn anything more. Was there a chance for some healing there? I wondered. Serious illnesses sometimes break good marriages. Sometimes they also mend broken ones. If the latter was going to prevail, it would not be the first time I had seen a major disease lead to reconciliation and healing of the deep wounds of lost love. Those things just seem to happen.

"Tell me, how do you react to perfumes and formaldehyde and tobacco smoke?" I changed the subject.

PSYCHONEUROIMMUNOLOGY: A GREAT ERROR

"What do you think of psychoneuroimmunology?" I asked Choua one day.

"Psychoneuroimmunology! Isn't that a jawbreaker of a word?" Choua smiled impishly. "But what does that mean?"

"It is the branch of medicine that deals with the interrelationships of the psyche, nervous system and immune system."

"Those mind-over-body gurus thrive on that, don't they?" Choua replied churlishly.

"It isn't just mind-over-body gurus," I replied. "Lots of

people in and out of the medical profession believe in the theory of mind-over-body healing."

"How ironic!" Choua spoke sternly that time. "It took you two centuries of medical philosophy and research to separate mind from body. It took you a near century to define the immune system as a system of antibodies and antigens—quite discrete from the brain and our psyche."

"It seemed to make sense then to separate the mind from the body," I remarked.

"And now you are devoting hundreds of millions of dollars to prove that the body and the mind indeed are interrelated. How could it have been any different? You physicians excel in reinventing the wheel, don't you?" Choua winked.

"What do you mean?" I asked, puzzled.

"Old Socrates, he had the last laugh."

"Why do you bring Socrates into this?" I asked, confused by Choua's reference to Socrates.

"Psychoneuroimmunology!" Choua chuckled. "The old man knew all about it."

"Socrates knew about psychoneuroimmunology?" I asked in disbelief. "I thought the term was coined during the last few decades."

"What do you think he meant when he said:

The great error of our day is this: Our physicians separate mind from body.

"Do you think Socrates knew about receptors on immune cells and about how some neurotransmitters link the workings of the brain and the immune system?" I asked.

"How did Tammy's immune system turn against her? What was the psychoneuroimmunology problem there?" Choua went on.

"You tell me."

"How did the loss of her mother lead to the formation of antibodies against the nuclei of her own cells—that's what ANA, antinuclear antibodies, are, aren't they?"

"Yes," I agreed.

"Eight years later, how did the threatened loss of her husband turn her immune system against her own myelin sheaths? Myelin sheaths are the insulation cover of nerves that normally prevent short-circuiting of electromagnetic impulses passing through the nerves. That is the essence of multiple sclerosis."

"Perhaps someday we will have a better understanding of the healing energy," I replied timidly. "Then we'll be able to answer your questions with the objectivity science demands."

"What did the death of Tammy's mother have to do with her developing lupus?" Choua pressed on. "What did her impending divorce have to do with her myelin sheaths? Why did Tammy's psychoneuroimmune dog bite her?"

"Stress depresses the immune system."

"Cells, molecules and electrons have their own intelligence, their own consciousness," Choua continued. "They *feel and respond*. As for the purist in science who feels a surging desire to ridicule me, I ask only that he observe individual cells shaved from living tissues and kept in tissue culture petri dishes. Observe and reflect upon the greater glory of the intelligence and consciousness of these cells. Reflect on how they adapt to their new life in the petri dish. See with awe the sheer energy of life."

"You are a poet," I teased him. "Yet I'm sure the skeptics in mainstream medicine will not be persuaded by your viewpoint."

"Oh yes, the skeptics in medicine!" Choua groused. "Why don't they reflect on the workings of the simple molecule of nitric oxide? It is made up of an atom of nitrogen and an atom of oxygen. Yet, it is a triumph of nature in molecular design, a marvel of biology."

"How does it work?"

"One of the simplest compounds known to us, nitric oxide is elegance in simplicity. It opens up the arteries thrown into spasms by adrenaline and breaks up cortical conspiracies."

"Do you mean it is an anti-stress molecule?"

"Tight arteries are tired arteries. They scream for help. An enzyme, nitric oxide synthase, acts upon the amino acid arginine and splits a molecule of nitric oxide, leaving behind molecules of another amino acid, citrulline. It is this simple molecule of nitric oxide that also serves as a messenger, whereby immune cells called phagocytes recognize and destroy foreign invaders like disease-causing bacteria and errant cells that cause cancer."

"Interesting ideas, but is all that scientifically valid?" I provoked him.

"Nitric oxide makes sense where nothing else does," Choua continued in earnest, ignoring my provocation. "It is produced by individual cells in time of need—without any commands from the thinking mind. Nitric oxide production is a local energy event. Each nitric oxide molecule, produced locally in response to a *local* need, dismantles the common belief that the mind-over-body approach heals."

"Is that sufficient to support your viewpoint that mind-over-body cannot work?" I prodded him.

"This simple molecule provides us a rational, scientifically sound and believable energetic-molecular mechanism to help us comprehend how autoregulation works in real life. It also helps explain why autoregulation does not work on some people for many months, and how it does work when finally it does. This molecule..."

"I don't follow that," I interrupted him.

"This molecule is one that holds the key to understanding how exhausted tissues can—and do—finally escape the cortical tunnels and walk into limbic openness," he continued without answering my question. "And, yes, it does open some windows to Sheila's suffering. And the suffering of Edward and Tammy. And of the suffering of all the other Sheilas, Edwards and Tammys. Nitric oxide, of course, is not a lone warrior rising against adrenergic tyranny. There are others. Some of them we know. Others, I am sure, will be recognized at some future time."

"Let's get back to nitric oxide. How does this fit into the notion that all molecular events are under control of genes?" I asked.

"Genes?" Choua frowned. "Why don't you bring genes into this? Genes do not control all events in biology any way."

"They don't?" I asked, surprised. "Will you name one that isn't."

"If genes control all events in life, what controls genes?"

"That's an interesting question," I admitted, then repeated my question. "Will you name one?"

"How do tiny microbes arrange themselves in intricate, yet consistent formations on culture plates?" he asked.

"I thought genes control that."

"Nop!" Choua chirped gleefully. "They certainly don't. The cover story of the July 6, 1995, issue of *Nature* was about secrets of self-organization in nature. Budrene and Berg of Harvard University reported how bacteria belonging to *E. coli* and *S. typhimurium* create complex, elaborate and highly symmetrical formation in cultures."

"How does that happen?"

"The microbes first produce aspartate, a simple molecule that serves as a chemical mover for bacteria—a chemotactant. Next, simple molecules such succinate and fumarate used as foods for microbes serve as an organizing influence. The final geometric patterns depend on initial conditions. The essential issue..."

"But, wait! You are drifting," I countered. "What do

geometric growth patterns of microbes have to do with what we are discussing? With nitric oxide and autoregulation?"

"The essential issue here," Choua continued, without acknowledging my question, "is that microbes not only produce simple molecules that organize them, they also *read* their micro-environment and respond accordingly. What the Harvard researchers call self-organization, at a fundamental level, is no different from your autoregulation. Self-organization in form is but a consequence of autoregulation in function." Choua nodded approvingly.

"I need to think about that," I said, then changed the subject. "Is there something we can do to stimulate nitric oxide?"

"Of course, there is!" Choua chuckled. "Don't you see it? Is that's the whole point of autoregulation—to cancel out the adrenergic molecular drive? To allow stressed and injured tissues to regain normal energy states in which molecules and cells can read their micro-environment and respond to them in appropriate way? Autoregulation, in its essence, is facilitating the natural principles of self-organization."

Choua stopped, stared at me with blank eyes for a few moments, then resumed,

ADRENERGIC MOLECULAR HYPERVIGILENCE

"One man gambles and his wife suffers from diarrhea. Another man fears he will lose his job after 25 years at his company and develops high blood pressure. A woman cares for her mother dying of cancer and suffers from unremitting pain. A salesman returns home without a sale, weary with fatigue. What is common in all these cases?"

"Stress, obviously," I replied.

"Right!" he grinned, then continued. "A young man suffers a sudden panic attack. He cannot breathe, has heart palpitations and thinks he is dying of a heart attack. A woman dashes into the street to yank away her toddler who is walking toward a speeding car. A lion chases a deer and the deer sprints to dodge the attacker. What are the molecular dynamics of these events? We glibly dismiss it as a stress reaction, the so-called fight or flight response. The role of adrenaline and its cousin molecules, catecholamines, in stress is well-known. They cause arteries in limbs and abdominal organs to tighten, muscles in the body to tense, pupils to dilate, heart rate to quicken, skin to rise in goose pimples, and the cortical brain to shift to a higher gear. Nature gave us this reaction for a survival advantage—so we can escape threats to life faster, or to dig our heels to fight out the aggressor. The problem is that these cortical molecular devices do not know their limits. Once triggered, they initiate cascade events, forever feeding upon themselves."

"The devices of the thinking mind?" I raised my eyebrows.

"Yes, cortical devices, in your autoreg lingo." Choua smiled. "The so-called chronic stress syndrome, of course, is nothing but adrenergic molecular hypervigilence. In this syndrome, the body organs are hit hard with a new stressor before they have a chance to recover from the previous insult. Relentless stress causes unrelenting demands on organs; the tissues scramble, suffer and finally suffocate. The role of many other neurotransmitters in the cause of other chronic disorders has also been explored in recent studies. The common thread in the energy dynamics in all these states is *cortical overdrive*. The question that has preoccupied me for some years is this: How do tissues counter cortical molecular hypervigilence? How do they escape from cortical torrents? How do they return to a limbic state? Do they do so because the cortical brain sends electromagnetic messages to them to ease up? Or do they send some neurotransmitters to cancel out the effects of adrenaline and its companion molecules—co-conspirators in cortical conspiracies? Or maybe individual cells in tightened arteries and spastic muscles have their own molecular devices to escape the tyranny of cortical tyrants?"

"How does an adrenergic dog bite?" I asked, bemused with Choua's choice of words.

"In the same way a teenager jolts his car on his first driving lesson. Easing off on the brake pedal and gently pressing on the gas pedal does not come naturally to him. Molecules have their own rhythms, their own timing, their own sense of space."

****

The general reader may wish to skip the text in the following eight pages (336 to 343) which relate my conversation with Choua about the complex concepts of turbulence and intermittency in physics. Choua believes these concepts are relevant to the matter of the bite of the gray dog—adverse energy response in the early stages of autoregulation. If so, please go to page 344.

DISORIENTED PHYSICS OF LIFE

"Do you know how humpback whales feed on schools of smaller fish?" Choua asked.

"How?" I asked.

"They build a net of bubbles to trap the fish before they engulf them," he explained.

"Nets of bubbles in the ocean?" I asked, puzzled.

"Humpbacks team up to hunt smaller fish. First, they find a school of small fish and dive deep into the ocean to position themselves below the fish. Then, all together, they swim up to the small fish in a spiral fashion, blowing air through their blow holes, creating a net of bubbles around the school of fish. The school of fish get totally disoriented by the walls of bubbles around them and cannot escape the open-mouthed whales as they shoot up to engulf their hapless victims."

"Why do the whales have to create bubble-nets to feed on smaller fish? Why can't they simply devour them?" I asked.

"Economy of effort," Choua elaborated. "Such communal bubble-netting allows the whales to collect more food with less effort."

"Why can't the prey swim through the bubbles?" I asked. "That shouldn't be difficult."

"They are disoriented by the physics of disorder," he grinned.

"Interesting! But what do bubble nets have to do with Sheila's neck spasms? Or with Edward's neck? Or with the bite of the gray dog?" I asked, puzzled.

"Disoriented physics of life!" Choua chuckled. "What is a

cunning hunting strategy—an economy of effort—for the whales is a wall of death for the prey."

"I still don't understand it. What do humpbacks have to do with negative energy responses to autoreg? What do bubbles have to do with the bite of the gray dog?" I persisted.

"Turbulence in the physics of biology!" he replied condescendingly.

"I don't understand," I admitted my confusion.

"Physics of life can be confusing," Choua spoke solemnly.

"Yeah, but I still don't understand what that has to do with the bite of the gray dog," I said, exasperated.

"It's really quite simple," Choua spoke softly. "I'll tell you a story."

"Another story?" I winced. "I haven't gotten the point of your previous stories. What makes you think this one will work?"

"Maybe this one will work." he winked.

ALL MY LIFE I HAVE HAD THINGS THROWN AT ME, THIS ONCE I COULDN'T TAKE IT

A grocer was alone in his shop. A thug entered the shop, looked around for a while, then walked over to the cash register, pulled a gun and demanded all the money in the cash register. The grocer turned pale and froze.

"Give me the money," the thug screamed at the grocer.

"Yes! No! Yes!" the grocer trembled as he looked at the video camera hung from the front door.

"Shut up! Hand me the money or I'll blow your brains out." The thug pointed the gun at the grocer's chest.

"Please, don't hurt me," the grocer pleaded urgently as he

recovered from the initial shock.

   With trembling hands, his delicate frame shaking uncontrollably, the grocer took out all the money from the cash register. The thug lunged toward the counter. Frightened out of his wits, the grocer threw all the money on the counter in front of the man. The thug hurriedly picked up the money, stared at the grocer for a few moments, then shot the grocer dead."
   "Why did he shoot the grocer?" I couldn't hold my curiosity. "He got all the money. Why did he kill the poor man?"
   "The thug was apprehended and tried days later," Choua continued, ignoring my question. "The prosecutor showed a video of the robbery in court. The jury was visibly shocked at the scenes of cold-blooded murder. It was an open and shut case. The thug admitted his crime. Predictably, the verdict was guilty. The judge retired for some time before pronouncing the punishment. When he returned to the court, the bailiff ordered the thug to stand up to hear the punishment for his crime. The judge looked at the thug with solemn eyes before speaking. 'Answer me,' he said to the thug, 'The frightened grocer didn't fight back. He didn't call for help. He didn't curse you. All he did was give you all the money. Why did you kill him?' The thug stayed motionless, his eyes downcast for several moments. Finally, he slowly raised his head, looked at the judge and replied, 'All my life, I have had things thrown at me. This once, I couldn't take it'."
   "A sad story with an unpredictable end," I remarked when Choua finished.
   "It can be the same for the gray dog. When the tissues are violated for years, their responses can be unpredictable."
   "Is that why you think the gray dog bit his master?" I asked in disbelief.
   "What do you think?" he laughed.
   "Do you really think that's what happens in autoregulation?

Things have been thrown at tissues for years. And they can take them no more."

"Turbulence in physics!" Choua's voice dropped suddenly and he fell silent.

THE ENZYME RESPONSES SOMETIMES OVERSHOOT THEIR MARK

"In simple terms," he began after several moments, "the bite of the gray dog represents enzyme functions in the healing response overshooting their mark."

"Explain that, Choua," I demanded.

"You know enzymes are catalysts—they make things happen in living beings."

"Yes."

"Enzymes are made up of proteins, and get easily oxidized and denatured."

"I agree."

"Injured enzymes are functionally impaired and cause unexpected, abnormal energetic-molecular responses. Thus, in autoregulation, the healing enzyme responses sometimes undershoot and the person feels no response from injured tissues. At other times, the injured enzymes overshoot their mark, creating unwanted, unpleasant responses."

"Is that what happened to the gray dog when he bit his master in confusion? His energy enzymes overshot their mark?" I asked.

"Yes. And that also explains why many of your very sick patients experience negative initial responses to autoregulation," he explained.

"Why do such negative responses disappear later?"

"Enzymes regenerate spontaneously during life. Ever so slowly, the injured enzymes are replaced with regenerated enzymes that function well. Also, the demands on enzymes are reduced as the person begins to heal."

"Some people told me they did autoregulation without any negative responses for months or years. Then they stopped meditation and self-regulation. When they became sick again and tried autoreg again, they experienced negative responses again. How do you explain that?" I asked.

"What's there to explain?" he asked. "The dynamics of the injury-healing-injury cycle are essentially the same. It doesn't matter much whether they occur for the first time or are repeated months and years later. As long as the fire of life burns, the simmering oxidative coals can turn into leaping oxidative fires as the total oxidative stress builds up."

Choua rubbed his temples, looked at the books on the shelves absently, then left the room.

TURBULENCE AND INTERMITTENCY

Choua returned after a few days. Without greeting me—as he frequently does when he visits me—he picked up a recent issue of *Nature* from my desk, opened it randomly and buried his head into its pages. It is one of his quirks. I have observed it for years, and it still amuses me. I looked at him for some moments, then returned to my microscope.

"I think I know why the thug shot the grocer," I said after

a while, "but I still don't understand why the gray dog bit his master."

"Doesn't the grocer's story explain that?" he asked, his head still buried in the pages of the journal.

"To be frank, Choua," I replied, "I really don't know what that grocer's story had to do with the bite of the gray dog. Or with Sheila's or John's problems. Or with initial negative energy responses in tissues, which many people experience with autoreg."

"And the wall of death that humpbacks create with their bubble nets?" Choua asked. "Does that explain something?"

"No," I replied curtly.

"Disoriented physics of life! Turbulence in physics!" Choua murmured.

"Please talk to me plainly, Choua," I pleaded. "Your stories don't explain it. Nor do I understand your oblique reference to turbulence in physics. Why should disoriented physics cause problems sometimes but not other times?"

"Perhaps it has something to do with what I'm reading now," Choua replied, his eyes still glued to the pages of *Nature*.

"What are you reading about?"

"Turbulence and intermittency in physics!" Choua finally looked up.

"Intermittency?" I asked, confused. "What is intermittency in physics?"

"Turbulence is unpredictability in life! Intermittency is nonlinearity in tissue energy dynamics!"

"You are answering puzzling questions with yet more puzzling answers. And that doesn't help," I protested.

"In fluid dynamics, turbulence is the unpredictable blend of order and disorder that occurs in fluid flows. It is a ubiquitous phenomenon according to this article," he closed the journal to look at the cover, "the March 30, 1995 issue of *Nature.*"

"I'm sorry, Choua," I shook my head in frustration. "I

can't relate any of that to cortical debraking—with bites of the gray dog," I persisted.

"Turbulence in physics of fluid dynamics measures the ratio of nonlinear inertial forces to the linear dissipative forces of friction within the fluid flow."

"Speak plainly to me, Choua," I pleaded. "Physics isn't my strength."

"Intermittency is pervasive in our world," he read from *Nature*, oblivious to my question. "Were the heavy car traffic in Bangkok not intermittent, pedestrians would be unable to cross the city's busy roads. Yet they cross these roads so frequently and so illegally that traffic lights have become irrelevant."

"So?" I asked, my confusion increasing.

"The article also says," Choua continued, closing the journal and looking at me for the first time since he entered my office, "that the same turbulence and intermittency occurs in financial markets where periods of trading frenzy are followed by quiescence. Furthermore, when one looks at these phenomena closely, one discovers that the periods of high volatility are themselves found to be made up of subperiods of relative quiet and bursts."

"What does all that have to do with cortical debraking?" I persisted.

"Such turbulence and intermittency has been discovered to affect water flow in rivers," he continued with his own preoccupation. "Two successive floods and two successive droughts of the river Nile were found to occur slightly more often than they should."

"But what do turbulence and intermittency in river flows have to do with..."

"The Nile's cycles of flood and drought," Choua cut me off, "imply an intermittency in time where years characterized mostly by flood are followed by years characterized mostly by droughts," Choua continued to read from *Nature*.

"I'll wait till you are finished with your physics gibberish," I groaned, exasperated.

"Both small- and large-scale turbulences are nonlinear —non-Gaussian," Choua grinned.

"So?" I protested.

"You write about visceral resistance—the difficulty some of your patients face in autoreg. The tissues don't respond. When they do, they overreact."

"But why?"

"Intermittency! That ubiquitous phenomenon in nature that blends order with disorder in ever-changing ways," Choua chugged along.

"Speak plainly, Choua, will you? What does turbulence in physics have to do with negative energy responses in autoreg?"

"Linear and predictable forces in nature are disrupted by nonlinear and unpredictable forces," Choua smiled disarmingly. "Then comes into play an intermittency in physics that restores some order but in ways quite distinct from the original order."

"Turbulence and intermittency! Is that your explanation of why the gray dog bites? Is that *your* theory?" I teased him.

"It is plausible, isn't it?" he grinned.

"Plausible, maybe. But is it factual?" I asked. "If it is true, then why does the gray dog bite repeatedly and eventually stop biting? Why do such individuals eventually succeed in autoreg and cease to experience the bites of the gray dog?"

"Intermittency brings the addictive behavior among disoriented neurons, and that works both ways." Choua grew serious.

LIFE IS NOT LINEAR

"Life isn't linear," Choua continued, "One plus one in biology doesn't always mean two. Sometimes, it means eleven. Biologic processes follow uneven, harmonic patterns—peaks and valleys! Biology isn't linear. Two and two don't always make four in biology—come to think of it, they almost never do. That's the nature of things. And that's where your problems begin."

"Yeah, so," I asked, unable to decipher Choua's logic.

"And when the troubled tissues respond, they overreact—what you call cortical debraking," Choua grinned.

"Yes, but I still don't know what they have to do with your turbulence and intermittency," I complained.

"Life is not linear," Choua repeated.

"You said that a few moments ago," I complained. "Are you saying the tissue responses in autoregulation are not linear?" I ventured a guess.

"Why should the physics of fluid dynamics in human tissues be any different than that in other living systems?" Choua asked the way teachers ask questions to little children.

"So the tissues under duress sometimes overshoot and sometimes undershoot! Is that it?" I guessed again.

"Turbulence and intermittency, I think, are very relevant to negative energy responses—to what you call visceral resistance and cortical debraking. Don't you agree?"

"Yes! No! Well, it isn't clear to me," I flustered.

"It is really quite simple," Choua grinned again. "You write a lot about simmering oxidative coals of anger and hostility, don't you? And how minor triggers fan those coals into leaping flames? Next, flames turn into raging fires, causing all forms of stress and disease in the various body organs. Right?"

"Right!" I replied timidly.

"Don't you see it is the same with simmering oxidative coals at neurotransmitter receptors and at neuromuscular conduction regions?" he gazed into my eyes. "Minor triggers evoke powerful negative responses. Simple thoughts of past slights and hurts fan the oxidative coals into bursts of fire. You do autoreg to free the injured tissues from the tyranny of the thinking mind. But before the cortical monkey yields, it delivers some parting kicks to the ailing tissues. You see, the monkey cannot help himself. The injured tissues are too bruised to slide smoothly into the quiet of the healing mode. They are jolted by turbulence. And..." Choua stopped in mid-sentence and rubbed his temple.

"And?" I pressed.

"Nonlinear dynamics is one of this century's most important scientific advance—the chaos theory, as it is popularly called. Do you know where the chaos theory came from?"

"Where?"

"Ecology!" he pouted. "Ecology was the cradle of the chaos theory. All ecologic models that have been studied to date are highly nonlinear in ways that admit possibilities of complex dynamics."

"Are you saying that the linear thinking in medicine—and linear models of treatment based on it—are not relevant to clinical care of the sick?" I asked, incredulous. "Even in acute, intensive medicine?"

"Why do you use intravenous injections of morphine in patients with life-threatening pulmonary edema?" he asked.

"Because it helps."

"What is the mechanism of action of morphine in acute pulmonary edema?"

"I don't think it is known."

"Isn't acute pulmonary edema an excellent example of your Fourth-of-July chemistry?"

"Yes," I confessed, then asked, "Do you think the Fourth-of-July chemistry of acute pulmonary edema is an example of the chaos theory in work?"

"Your autoregulation works the same way as morphine—it puts out the chaotic oxidative fireworks of your Fourth-of-July chemistry. But..."

"But what?" I interrupted him impatiently.

"The energy pulses in injured tissues misfire initially—just like the gray dog," he continued calmly. "Sheila's neck muscles go into spasms. Edward suffers the agony of someone turning and twisting his neck, yanking it through the ceiling. Don't you see it all fits with the phenomenon of turbulence—the phenomenon that blends disorder with order."

"Why did Sheila's painful muscle spasms subside? Why did Edward get better?" I asked.

"Intermittency! That brings some order back into disorder created by turbulence. Don't you see it all fits?" he beamed.

"But are you sure?" I expressed doubt.

"Sure of what?" he seemed irked by my question.

"Are you sure?" I asked, "that the piece in *Nature* really applies to changes I see during autoregulation?"

"I..." Choua stopped in mid-sentence, stared at me for a few moments. "I don't know, *silly.*" Choua grinned churlishly and walked out.

There is a cortical monkey in each of us. Most of us see him clearly. Also, there is a gray dog in each of us. Many of us are totally oblivious of his existence.

Every Wednesday I give autoregulation training to a group of four or five new patients and several who return for second or third training sessions. I hear the moans of the gray dog from one or two patients in almost each group. Fortunately, the bite of the gray dog is not as bad for most people as it was for Sheila, Edward and Tammy. Most people experience spasms in their neck muscles, low back stiffness, mild chest discomfort, anxiety, rapid heart rate, lightheadedness and occasional episodes of watering or searing eyes. Such bites are brief and of no consequence. All a person has to do to overcome them is to persist in autoregulation.

It seems improbable that man will ever fully understand the healing energy of love, or to be more precise, the healing energy of God. Medical technology, itself an expression of God's energy, is beginning to allow us to measure some things about love and then reproduce them. Measurement and reproducibility make up the language of science. One day, it seems to me, the men of medicine and men of spirits will meet at some summit of union. The energy of love will have brought them together.

The Cortical Monkey and Healing

Chapter 10

The Thinking Ants

Just because one can see a question define itself, one isn't entitled to its answer.

One day I saw Ronald K., a young man who suffered from disabling chronic fatigue. Like other chronic fatigue sufferers —human canaries as I call them—Ronald enumerated a long list of troubling symptoms. He kept reciting descriptions of brain fog, loss of memory, numbness, muscle twitching and other nervous symptoms. At one point Ronald broke down and said,

I'm tortured by this red hot nail that somebody keeps constantly driving into my head. Dr. Ali, please believe me, it's like my brain is being zapped with a million volts—10, 15, 20 times a day. None of the previous doctors I saw could explain it. Can you?

The problem, of course, is not that I don't understand the cause of such unbearable suffering. The challenge for me is how to explain to the Ronalds of this world in a language they can easily understand the true nature of oxidative injury to their molecules and cells. Oxidation is the loss of electrons, the tiniest, subatomic energy particles. In simple language, oxidation is the loss of energy by high-energy molecules so that they become lower-energy molecules. People like Ronald need to learn how oxidation violates their brain cells—how their neurotransmitters are blocked, how their cell receptors are mutilated, and how the electromagnetic charges on their cell membranes are disrupted.

Chronically ill persons need to understand that oxidation damages their blood cells and clots blood plasma proteins. Oxidation cooks—figuratively and literally—the body's molecules and cells. They need to know that accelerated oxidative injuries—oxidative fires in my terminology—destroy to varying degrees all their body tissues. The oxidative fires are ignited and fanned by undiagnosed allergies; environmental pollutants and toxic metals; viruses, bacteria, yeasts, and parasites in their blood and various other body organ ecosystems; and by the unrelenting stress of modern life and sickness. All those factors create a Fourth-of-July chemistry under their skin which further fans the oxidative fires in their bodies.

Symptoms such as 'being zapped with a million volts' do not exist in medical texts because the texts are written by people who are still wedded to nineteenth-century notions of diseases and drugs. That's the main reason why mainstream physicians simply dismiss the agonizing symptom-complexes, such as those described by Ronald and other human canaries, as "all-in-the-head." Then, tragically, patients like Ronald are referred to psychiatrists.

I usually respond to anguished inquiries such as that made by Ronald by performing my MOST test (microscopic oxidative stress test) with a drop of blood taken from the tip of the patient's finger. I use a high-resolution microscope equipped with phase-contrast, dark-field optics for this purpose. The microscopic images are projected on a video screen so that a magnification order of ten to fifteen thousand or more is achieved. I can then observe—and effectively demonstrate to the patient—the nature and extent of oxidative injury to blood elements, as well as the presence of microbes in the blood.

I looked at Ronald's pale face. His sad eyes searched mine for an answer to his question. I told him that the MOST test might give us some clues. With that I pricked the tip of his right index finger, drew a drop of blood, prepared a thin smear, put the slide on the microscope stage and began to study the magnified images. Ronald bolted up from his slumped position and leaned to the video screen for a closer look.

"You have two visitors," Choua spoke as I focused my microscope.
"Who?" I asked, looking up.
"Two ants."
"Where?" I scanned the surface of my desk, looking for insects.
"You can't see them, Mr. Pathologist," Choua chuckled.
"Oh, that," I mumbled, a trifle embarrassed. "Another one of those Choua pranks. What next?"
"The ants think it's a miracle."
"What's a miracle?" I asked.
"They watched you draw a drop of blood from Ronald's fingertip, make a smear on a slide, turn on the microscope and see many images on the video screen. They think it's a miracle."
"It isn't a miracle, just a microscope attached to a video screen."
"The images of Ronald's blood enchant them. They've never seen anything like it. You shine a light through a drop of blood and pictures of a thousand bodies appear on the video screen, turning, twisting, bumping into each other."
"That's good. I'm glad my work entertains your visiting ants," I said and began to record my microscopic findings.

Ronald's blood smear was "dirty"—strewn with dead and dying cells everywhere in the field of blood plasma. Some other cells were damaged, deformed or sludged. I focused on the few cells that appeared healthy, and compared them with those that were badly damaged. I explained to Ronald that smooth-surfaced cells that floated singly in the pool of his plasma were healthy, like fresh cherries. The clumped and deformed cells had been damaged by oxidant stress and were like stale cherries with cracked skin that stuck to each other. Oxidant stress, I explained, had been caused by undiagnosed and untreated allergies, pollutants and microbes. Furthermore, just as the cells in his blood were injured by oxidant stress, so were those in his brain. Finally, I explained that those 'million volts zapping' his head came from nerve cells that misfired incessantly as they were continually violated.

Next, I focused on the yeast organisms that moved around singly and in small clusters, evidencing oxidative damage to blood plasma proteins. Slowly and in simple words, I explained to Ronald the abnormalities I noted in his blood smear and why his damaged cells and proteins were the cause of his symptoms.

OXIDATIVE COALS CURDLE BLOOD: THE BEGINNING OF OXIDATIVE COAGULOPATHY

"My ants are very impressed with your explanation," Choua continued.

"Please tell them how grateful I am for their comments," I replied in jest.

"In some places, the blood plasma appears condensed. The ants want to know why."

"Those are congealed plasma proteins."

"What causes them to congeal?"

"The oxidative stress that damages cell membranes also damages plasma proteins—literally cooks them. Plasma congeals when its soluble protein, fibrinogen, is oxidatively converted into insoluble protein, fibrin. That's how the blood plasma thickens."

"And the thin flakes that float amid the congealed plasma?"

"When oxidative injury advances, fibrin threads trap blood platelets and the congealed plasma thickens."

"And those lumpy floaters?"

"Your visiting ants want to know a lot, don't they?" I asked in good humor. "Well, you tell them I call those lumpy floaters microclots because that's precisely what they are—clotted lumps of blood proteins, enzymes and hormones."

"What's the significance of microclots in circulating blood?"

"That's big trouble. Those microclots are simmering coals that cause yet more oxidative injury to the cells and plasma proteins that surround them."

"They create a chain reaction, is that it?"

"Yes."

"If it's such a dangerous chain reaction, why doesn't it cause death?"

"Because there are other proteins in the blood that dissolve or digest microclots, freeing up capillaries and restoring circulation. The system of fibrin-dissolving proteins is called the fibrinolytic system."

"Aha! So microclots dissolve in circulating blood as new ones form. Tell me, what would happen if the fibrinolytic system was sluggish and more microclots were formed than were dissolved?"

I peered into Choua's eyes and tried to decipher what was

on his mind. Who are his ants? Why did he bring them into my study of Ronald's blood? Of course, I'm familiar with Choua's pranks and his schizophrenic flight of ideas by now. I knew his visiting ants had some sort of message for me. But what? Something about Ronald's blood morphology, or was it about something altogether different? I knew that just because Choua had begun with his ants' interest in the MOST test didn't mean that's where he would end.

I wondered about his ants while I moved the slide to scan several fields on the video screen and settled on an area that displayed a large, thick deposit of amorphous material that nearly filled the screen. Within and surrounding the large deposit were visible yeast organisms.

"What's that?" Choua inquired, pointing to the deposit.

"Tell your ants that is how microclots grow when mycotoxins and other types of toxins cause the blood proteins to clot. The proteins curdle, so to speak, at a rate that far exceeds the ability of fibrin-dissolving proteins to clear them."

"That's like the bloodstream being on fire. Fascinating! Blood curdling isn't a medically acceptable term. Why don't you call it oxidative coagulopathy?"

"*Oxidative coagulopathy*! Choua, did you just make that up?" I asked with a laugh, then added. "Not a bad name for the process."

"I think so. You'll have much better luck with oxidative coagulopathy than with blood curdling. Your colleagues will agree that it is a good term to refer to what you're describing. I mean the oxidative clotting of proteins of the blood and lymph plasmas, as well as of proteins of cell and plasma membranes of subcellular organelles. Isn't that what you're really talking about?"

"Yes, well, no. It's not just proteins. I mean..."

"I know. I know it isn't just proteins," he didn't let me finish. "Oxidative injury also oxidizes and denatures fats and sugars of blood plasma and cell membranes. But my term oxidative coagulopathy is better than your blood curdling, isn't it? Isn't that how it really all begins at energetic-molecular-cellular levels? Tell me, what happens next?"

"Continuing oxidative injury causes yet more damage to proteins, fats and sugars. Microclots enlarge, coalesce and form large ugly curdles. I call them micro-plaques. Those plaques comprise cooked proteins, dead and dying cells, dead and dying yeasts, bacteria, and God knows what other junk."

"What's the clinical significance of micro-plaques?"

"They're more dangerous than thin, wooly microclots."

"Why?"

"Because the thin microclots can be dissolved but thick micro-plaques apparently can't. So they have a greater capacity for clogging capillaries and suffocating tissues. They're bigger, hotter coals than microclots that burn blood cells and plasma proteins more efficiently. If that's not checked, it turns into DIC —disseminated intravascular coagulation."

"Isn't DIC considered a fatal condition by mainstream doctors?"

"Yes, DIC is considered potentially fatal unless it's controlled quickly," I replied.

"See, that's why you should accept my term. The use of oxidative coagulopathy will distinguish it from DIC and keep you out of trouble with your colleagues in mainstream medicine."

"But my blood curdling is also very dangerous if it goes unchecked. It can..."

"I know! I know!" Choua cut me off. "I know it's the same thing, but don't you want to stay out of trouble with mainstreamers? Don't you think you've caused enough problems for yourself by now? You call oxidative coagulopathy DIC and you will never hear the end of it. Haven't they called you a quack enough times?"

I suppressed a smile and said nothing.

LEAKY CELL MEMBRANE SYNDROME

"My ants want to know about damage done to blood cells in oxidative coagulopathy," Choua resumed.

"They are curious little beings, aren't they? They must have overgrown heads," I mocked.

"Why do Ronald's red blood cells get sludged?" he asked, oblivious to my tone.

"Oxidative injury cooks proteins and fats in their cell membranes and changes their surface charges. Also it pokes holes in them, making them leaky and sticky," I replied.

"The leaky cell membrane syndrome. That's neat! Isn't that one of your terms?"

"Yes," I nodded. "With cell membranes shot full of holes, what's inside the cells hemorrhages out, and what's outside floods in. Tell your info-hungry ants that that's how cells become deficient in magnesium, potassium, molybdenum and taurine. That's also how cell innards are flooded with excess calcium, which poisons cell enzymes."

"That's good stuff. My ants like it. What happens next?"

"The damaged cells become angulated and spinous, and that impairs their flow within the capillaries. When that happens, the cells cannot transport oxygen and nutrients."

"Why do blood platelets get clumped?"

"For the same reason, Choua. For the same reason," I

replied, a trifle annoyed at his repetitious inquiries. "Your clever ants should be able to deduce something that simple. Free radicals that cause oxidative injury to blood proteins and plasma also oxidize fats and phospholipids in blood platelets, making them sticky and causing them to clump. Of course, that further fans the fires of oxidative coagulopathy."

"The ants are impressed. They think the whole thing is nothing less than a miracle."

Choua smiled cryptically. What's that about? I wondered. What are his ants up to? Choua had watched me do the MOST test for other patients on several occasions. He had heard me explain to my patients things I saw on the video. I began to doubt that his ants were interested only in blood. There had to be other things. But what? I looked at him. He seemed lost in his own thoughts.

THE KILLER YEAST HUNT DOWN WEAKENED IMMUNE CELLS

"What is that rod-like structure?" Choua broke the silence, pointing to a bacterium that appeared on the video screen.

"You know that's a bacterium, don't you?" I asked, irritated at his pretense.

"Is that normal?" he asked, oblivious to my irritation. "I mean, should you see microbes floating in the blood like that?"

"Yes. No, well it isn't that simple," I faltered.

"Why not?" Choua's eyes narrowed.

"Because everyone has some bacteria floating in the blood. Their mere presence doesn't signify a disease."

"Then why did you say yes and no?"

"Because in this blood smear there are too many of them, and the leukocyte immune cells seem sluggish."

"Why are leukocyte immune cells sluggish?"

"What do your ants really want from me, Choua?" I complained.

"Actually, the ants are very impressed. So much information from just one drop of blood! Tell them, why are those leukocyte immune cells sluggish?"

"In the early stages of invasion of the bloodstream by microbes, the immune cells gear up to gobble the invaders. They show signs of activation, and their digestive granules move around actively within them. Later, when they are overwhelmed by waves of microbes, they're made sluggish—even paralyzed—by microbial toxins," I explained.

"What are those round, white bodies?" he asked, pointing to one video field.

"Yeast."

"Oh! What are they doing there?"

"Yeast have as much right as anything else to be in the blood, don't they?" I shot back.

"Where do they come from?" he asked evenly.

"From the bowel."

"My ants want to know if they have anything to do with Ronald's brain being zapped with a million volts?"

"I know your ants want to know everything. But, seriously, Choua, what do your ants really want to tell me. I think their interest in Ronald's blood is just a prelude to something else. Is it about yeasts? Or is it about something altogether different?"

"The ants want to know how Ronald gets zapped with a million volts." He sidestepped my questions.

"Okay, have it your way." I sighed. "There's an interesting observation I made some time ago. If you keep observing a yeast organism floating in fluid plasma over a period of a few hours, it causes clotting of plasma proteins around it. Sometimes I see amazing things. The yeast organisms invade the weakened immune cells, grow within them and cause them to explode. Then they're free to poison and kill yet other immune cells."

"Then what?" Choua's eyes widened.

"Patients who die of chemotherapy almost always show yeast overgrowth and infections. That's one way it all ends."

"Frightening, isn't it?" he shivered. "Tell me, how do clotted proteins in the blood cause a million volts zapping in the brain?"

"Plasma microclots in the circulating blood act as simmering coals, lighting up a thousand fires wherever they go. That's what they do in the brain. That's how yeast, microbes, microclots, and micro-plaques cause so many problems of mood, mentation, and memory. So many patients live in a fog, others are tortured by electric sparks like those Ronald experiences."

"Do you ever see protein microclots in the circulating blood of healthy patients?"

"Yes, but infrequently and in much smaller numbers."

"What happens to protein microclots in the end?"

"They are dissolved by certain enzymes in the normal plasma—the proteolytic enzymes."

"Why can't those proteolytic enzymes dissolve protein microclots in Ronald's blood?"

"Because there are simply too many microclots there."

"The oxidative fireworks. It cooks up more protein microclots than the proteolytic enzymes can break up. Is that it?"

"That's it. Tell me, are your ants now satisfied?"

"Didn't I tell you they are very impressed by you? I mean they were impressed even when they didn't know what all those blood pictures meant. Now they are overwhelmed."

"May I be introduced to them now?" I mock-pleaded.

"First, the ants want to know how you learned all that

about oxidative injury to blood cells, plasma proteins, bacteria and yeast."

"It took me long hours of microscopic study of blood morphology. Tell your ants I have been a student of medicine now for about 40 years. All those years of hard work went into making sense of what viruses and parasites do to the human ecosystems. And how good nutritional status of the patient helps him fight off such infections, and how poor nutrition makes the immune cells vulnerable."

Choua fell silent and gazed at my desk. I followed his gaze to a blank slide by the microscope. I waited for him to resume.

ECOTOXINS, MYCOTOXINS, METABOLIC TOXINS AND OXIDATIVE SYNDROMES

"Ronald also suffers from fibromyalgia. My ants are curious if you know what causes fibromyalgia and other types of muscle pain," Choua spoke finally.

"That's simple. It's all oxidative injury. Sludged cells, clumped platelets, and micro-plaques clog the tiny capillaries in the muscles and choke the tissues. Then ecotoxins, mycotoxins, and metabolic toxins including lactic acid accumulate in the muscles. There, they cause muscle spasms and create tender, painful trigger points. Of course, all those toxins cause further damage to cells and plasma proteins, triggering new cycles of clogged capillaries and spastic blood vessels and yet more accumulation of toxins and yet more muscle pain syndromes."

"How about skin pain?"

"The same mechanism. Oxidative injury damages blood

cells and plasma proteins, forming microclots that cause spasms that choke off blood vessels. The skin becomes cold, sensitive to the touch and painful."

"And the pain of arthralgia and arthritis?"

"Oxidative injury to the synovium, the joint lining and the muscles surrounding the joints."

"And digestive problems in the stomach?"

"Why should that be any different? It's the same oxidative injury. Acid-producing cells in the stomach begin to misfire and pour out excess acid that chews up the stomach lining."

"Why do your human canaries so often complain of poor digestion? Why do they say their food just sits in their stomachs?"

"Because ecotoxins and mycotoxins also make the stomach muscle sluggish—sometimes even paralyze it. Then the food just sits there."

"And heart palpitations and skipped beats?"

"Sugar-insulin-adrenaline roller coasters that unleash oxidative storms in the heart muscle. The same oxidative injury violates the nerves in the heart, making them jittery."

"Many patients with severe fatigue and other immune disorders experience visual difficulties. Sometimes they can't see clearly for hours. What causes that?"

"That's not hard to understand. There's only one retinal artery supplying the visual fields in the eyes. If a microclot or a micro-plaque occludes that artery or causes the artery to go into intense spasms, the patient can't see until the microclot dissolves and the arterial spasms resolve."

"My ants can't believe how you make everything look so simple and easy."

"This isn't about Ronald's blood at all, is it, Choua? What do your ants really want to say? What do *you* want them to say? Why don't you speak plainly?" I complained forcefully.

Choua grinned, then rubbed his temples. I waited.

"The ants were a little skeptical. They wanted me to assure them that what you claim to be scientifically sound, it is actually so."

"Tell them those are my microscopic observations. I don't know what others will think of them," I replied curtly.

"Right! Right!" Choua chirped, ignoring my growing irritation. "The ants know true science is purity of observation."

"Thanks for that vote of confidence," I said sarcastically.

"That's okay," he went on condescendingly. "Would you now tell them about the detoxification processes in the liver?" he asked.

"The same oxidative stuff, Choua. Excess ecotoxins, mycotoxins, bacterial toxins, and metabolic toxins overload the liver enzyme detoxification system, so the liver begins to fail."

"My ants challenge that glib answer. They think if that were really true, mainstream doctors would diagnose liver injury in their patients with chronic fatigue syndrome."

"The problem is that mainstream doctors don't do the right tests. There are sensitive tests for that purpose, but they don't know about them either."

"What other tests?"

"Please inform your info-starved ants that increased urinary levels of D-glucaric acid indicate that oxidative enzymes in the liver are working overtime to detoxify eco- and mycotoxins. Increased urinary levels of mercapturic acid mean that the liver is losing a lot of glutathione in the detoxification process."

"The ants are grateful for that lesson in chemistry." Choua smiled, evidently enjoying himself at my expense. "Chronic fatiguers—your human canaries—often look dehydrated. Why?"

"Oxidant stress creates an excess of metabolic toxins. And, of course, mycotoxins and ecotoxins, which caused the accelerated oxidative molecular injury in the first place, add to the total burden on the kidneys. The kidneys try hard to rid the body of that toxic overload by excreting it with water, so the patient gets dehydrated."

"Why do they break out in rashes?"

"The lungs are the most cost-effective waste organs of the body. What they cannot clear, the kidneys try to clear. When both organs cannot cope, the skin tries to act like a waste organ."

"How does the skin function like a waste organ?"

"That's the problem. It begins to erupt."

"Wow! Who told you that?"

"My patients' skin."

"Neat! Neat!" Choua exclaimed. "The ants love it. Tell them about the kidneys."

"Kidneys try to do their best to rid the body of the toxic overload, but there's a limit. They lose essential minerals, salt and bicarbonate ions. The chronically ill are always dehydrated unless they drink a gallon or more of water every day and take supplemental sea salt."

"What else?"

"Poor circulation will give them cold hands and feet and might cause skin soreness and pain."

"What else?"

"Poor circulation in the bowel will cause maldigestion and malabsorption, with bloating, flatulence and cramps."

"What else?"

"Choua, the oxidative fires in the circulating blood can affect any and all body organs."

"Is that why human canaries experience strange symptoms referable to all body organs?"

"Yes. At least, that's my view."

"Do most doctors recognize how ecotoxins and mycotoxins cause microclots in plasma proteins? Do they know how microclots and micro-plaques float in the circulating blood like smoldering coals, igniting oxidative fires wherever they travel?"

"I don't know about others, but I'm telling you things that I've observed myself and conclusions that I've drawn from them."

"What do you think drug doctors will say when they hear about your theory of mycotoxins causing microclots and micro-plaques and about clots and plaques causing all those weird symptoms?"

"I think they'll agree with me when, and if, they ever study the blood of human canaries the way I have."

"What do your patients think when they see their damaged blood ecosystem on the video screen?"

"They seem relieved. It means a lot to them when someone can objectively show them what's wrong with them at molecular and cellular levels. The microscopic images are revealing and relieving. Sometimes, my grown-up patients break down and cry like babies when they see that they're not losing their minds—only their blood cells and plasma proteins."

"Mainstream doctors often refer chronic fatigue patients to psychiatrists. What do you think of that?"

"What do your ants think of that?" I asked back.

"Ludicrous! The ants thinks that's ludicrous," he growled. "The ants think it's pathetic how psychiatrists never try to learn what really hurts human canaries. The ants have no patience for frivolous psychiatric theories, they respect only facts."

"Enlightened beings, your ants, aren't they?" I taunted.

"The ants want to know if you can diagnose cancer from a drop of blood."

"Of course, some cancers, such as leukemia, are readily diagnosed by MOST because you can see the malignant cells in the circulating blood. Other types of cancers, however, are not directly seen. But patients with cancer often show peculiar patterns of microclot and micro-plaque formation."

"Those ants are smitten by you. They're astounded by how much you can tell about a patient simply by looking at a drop of blood. They want to know how you became so wise."

"Me, wise?" I tried not to blush. "There's really nothing astounding there. Anyone with this type of microscope and experience can make those observations."

"Anyone can observe all that." A far away look appeared in Choua's eyes. He looked out the window, then repeated, "Anyone can observe all that. Then why don't they?"

I braced myself for some surprise turn by Choua. I knew it was overdue. Choua doesn't engage in volleys of questions like that without something on his mind. He had obviously set the stage for something. The ants were his characters. But what was he on to? Moments passed, then he spoke:

MIRACLES OF MICROSCOPY

"The ants want to understand the miracle of microscopy. They want to know everything that you know."

"*Everything* I know?" I asked in good humor. "How much time do they have?"

"That's the problem. They have errands to run and can't stay here for more than five minutes."

"Let me understand that, Choua. Your visiting ants want me to teach them *everything* I know about medicine, but they have only *five* minutes to spare. Is that it?"

"I know it may be a little awkward for you. My ants know it too. But they do want to understand the miracle of microscopy, and they realize they'll need to know as much as you do for that."

"Choua, please let *their antnesses* know that I've been a student of medicine for 40 years. It took me that many years to learn what I know. Now they insist that I transmit all that knowledge to them in five minutes! Is that the proposition?"

"Yeah," he replied seriously, then grinned. "That's about it. But the ants know you believe in miracles. Don't you?"

I didn't know how to respond. I covered my face with my hand, then rubbed my head. We were silent for some minutes.

FLOUR, HONEY, YEAST AND ANTS

"Alyson Hamilton, our nurse at the Blairstown office, told me something interesting about ants the other day," I finally spoke.

"What?" Choua asked absent-mindedly.

"She told me that she read some place about a natural remedy for coping with carpenter ants. You prepare a mixture of flour, honey, and yeast and sprinkle it wherever you find carpenter ants."

"Huh! A mixture of flour, honey and yeast. What does that do?"

"The ants feast on the yeast mixture. Once inside the ants' stomachs, the yeast feasts on the mixture of honey and flour and produces a lot of baby yeast, and together they cause a lot of fermentation and gas."

"So the ants' bellies bloat and they suffer bellyache. Is that it?"

"Well, that's not all. The yeast don't simply stop at bloated bellies. They continue to multiply, producing mycotoxins that make the ants sick. Finally, when there is enough fermentation and gas, it explodes the ants' bellies, killing them."

"Why did you tell me that?" he asked sternly.

"I thought what Alyson told me was funny. I thought you might find it funny too."

"You're an ant," he said.

"I'm an ant?" I asked, caught by his unexpected pronouncement.

"Yes, you're an ant," he repeated indifferently.

"Okay, so I'm an ant," I sighed. "I should have known better. I'm sorry. I shouldn't have brought up Alyson's story about flour, honey and yeast."

"I'm an ant," he continued.

"You too? I'm relieved." I laughed. "That means there are four of us ants here now, though I haven't had the honor of being formally introduced to your visiting ants."

"All of us are ants." Choua said solemnly.

"Pray, tell me, what led you to such a sweeping conclusion?" I asked, taunting.

"My ants irked you because they had the audacity to ask you to teach them medicine."

"They wanted to know everything—and all in *five* minutes! Your ants have overgrown heads and swollen brains, don't they?"

"Their heads are no more overgrown and their brains no more swollen than human ants," he deadpanned.

"What? Who are human ants? What are you rambling about?"

"People who deny miracles simply because they don't understand how miracles might work. You say my ants have overgrown heads because they ask you too many questions. Right?" Choua chimed.

"Right. No, well. I mean, that's not the point," I faltered. "Your ants or human ants, it's preposterous for anyone to think they can learn medicine in just five minutes."

"Preposterous?" Choua's forehead furrowed. "Tell me, what is more preposterous? My ants who want to learn everything in medicine in five minutes or your human ants who claim they can know everything in nature in one life time?"

"You're nuts!" I shouted.

"Why do you think my ants who want to learn MOST in five minutes are more stupid than your human ants who want to learn about miracles in just as much time?" he gored.

"You're crazy!" I didn't know whether to laugh or scream.

"Why is it less stupid for the human ants to insist that they fully understand the workings of the higher *presence* than it is for the insect ants to insist they fully understand the workings of the human body?"

"Oh God! You're schizoid today."

"Don't you see the obvious: your mind is your nemesis. When you deny miracles, you..."

"I don't deny miracles," I interrupted him. "And..."

"Only the profoundly ignorant deny miracles," he didn't let me finish.

"I remember you told me that before."

"You mock my ants. You think they have overgrown heads because they ask too many questions about blood morphology. You tell me they have swollen brains because they are eager to learn everything in medicine and claim they could do it faster than you. But you don't see the obvious. Your gurus of drug medicine—your human ants—insist that miracles cannot happen just because they cannot be reproduced in their controlled studies. Don't you see how ludicrous that is?"

"What are you ranting about?" I asked, baffled by his reference to controlled studies.

"You tell me my ants have overgrown heads and swollen brains. Don't you see your human ants also have overgrown heads and swollen brains? Only their heads aren't overgrown with wisdom, but with arrogance of pseudoscience of drugs. Your human ants also have swollen brains—swollen with the edema of hubris, not with understanding of the miracles of the healing phenomena."

"What's you eating you, Choua?" I asked, exasperated.

Choua stared at me, then turned and looked out the window.

TO KNOW A MIRACLE, YOU HAVE TO GO PAST THE MIND

"Okay, let's have it, Choua. What's on your mind?" I asked. "My head is heavy, and I'm not at all clear about where this conversation about blood clots, yeast and ants is taking us."

"We're all ants with overgrown heads and swollen heads—our skulls are too big for our tails."

"Okay. What else?" I prodded.

"You worship your mind because you think it can create. You believe you are clever because you can think—you invent things because you consider yourself inventive. You claim you are superior merely because you consider other living beings inferior. You mocked my ants because all along you thought they were really not there. No sir! You wouldn't talk to mere ants."

"Wait! Wait," I yelled. "The ants didn't ask me any questions. You did! How could I talk to them directly? Those snobbish little beasts didn't bother to even reveal themselves to me."

"There! You prove my point," he burst into laughter.

I was both perplexed and annoyed at Choua's pranks—as well as at my myself for calling his ants snobbish beasts. I shook my head and found myself laughing as well.

"You're obsessed with searching for the *absolute* truth because you presume you're entitled to it," Choua resumed. "Your colleagues dismiss miracles because miracles cannot be double-blinded and crossed over. You talk about rules and regulations of *spirituality* as if you know anything about spirituality. You write about laws of spiritual success. Isn't that a farce? Tell me, why would the ancients speak about the mind-body-spirit trio if not to admit that the spiritual was beyond the reach of their physical senses as well as the reach of the mind—beyond their bodies and their minds?"

"Is that your point of view, or are the ants speaking through you?" I asked caustically.

"Don't you see that whatever *can* be experienced with the physical senses or perceived by the mind cannot be spiritual?" he went on, ignoring my question. "For the spiritual to be discrete from the body and the mind, it must be beyond the reach of either. One cannot reach the spiritual by seeing, smelling, or hearing—or by superior thinking. Indeed, if that were not true, there would be no need for the trio. Mind-body duo would have been enough."

"Are we talking about miracles or spirituality?" I tried to follow his line of reasoning.

"The spiritual and miracles are the same thing. The problem is with the mind. It can think only about what it knows. Newton said that if there were no other proof of the existence of God, he would look at his thumb and know He exists. What did he mean by that?"

"Why don't you ask your ants?" I teased.

"Einstein said when a person cannot surrender to the mysterious, he is as good as dead. What did he mean?"

"Your ants probably know about that as well."

"Picasso said that when he went to the woods he had something green in his stomach. He painted to get rid of that green. What did he mean?"

"I don't know."

"How long have you been looking at blood smears with your microscope?"

"Many years."

"Do you sometimes see things in those blood smears that you never saw before?"

"That happens sometimes."

"When did you first recognize blood plasma curdles in blood smears?"

"Several years ago when I began to use my Bradford microscope with high-resolution, bright-light, phase-contrast and dark-field optics."

"Did you ever dissect coronary arteries blocked by plaques at autopsy during the last fifteen years?"

"Of course, yes. Many times. Why do you ask?"

"And you did that in dead bodies in the morgue downstairs while you examined living blood cells in the laboratory upstairs?"

"Yes. But what's the point of all that?" I asked, irritated.

"Tell me, how could you look at plasma microclots in blood smears and at the same time dissect occluded coronary arteries year after year and not recognize something quite obvious?" He ignored my irritation.

"What?" I asked, puzzled. "What is that something quite obvious which I failed to recognize?"

"When did you first suspect that the blood plasma curdles you saw in peripheral blood smears were the beginning of coronary artery disease?"

"Only recently."

"When did you first publish your theory of spontaneity of

oxidation?"

"Over fifteen years ago."

"If you recognized that oxidative injury was the true mechanism of tissue injury in *all* diseases over fifteen years ago, why did it take you so long to see the link between the plasma curdles produced by oxidative injury and coronary artery disease?"

"Why?" I asked baffled. "I don't know why. I guess I never thought about it," I replied lamely.

"How could you not see something that evident for so many years?" he pressed.

"Something require more time to reveal themselves. Sometimes it takes a long time to see simple things."

"*Some things require more time to reveal themselves.*" He repeated after me slowly, emphasizing each word. "How do things reveal themselves?"

"I don't know! I don't know," I replied, exasperated. "What's the matter with you, Choua?"

"Just curious," he replied with a smirk.

"You engage in some nutty conversations, but this one is nuttier than most. To tell you the truth, I've a headache now just listening to you," I complained.

"Some headaches have their benefits." Choua chuckled. "Do you know how Greek goddess, Athena, was born?"

"No," I replied curtly. "And, to be candid, I don't care for a lesson in Greek mythology right now."

"Zeus, the Greek supergod, once had a splitting headache," he went on, ignoring my protest. "Then a miracle happened. His head split and out came the goddess Athena in full splendor—wrapped in her gold-colored, embroidered velvet robe laced with precious stones, and her glittering crown. Once Athena emerged, Zeus's skull wound closed spontaneously and his headache subsided." Choua laughed out loud.

"Would you cut it out, Choua," I snapped.

"Who knows what might come out of your headache?" Choua bared his teeth in a smile.

"You're nuts!" I blurted, then broke out laughing. "Tell me, Choua, what do Newton and Einstein have to do with Zeus? What does Picasso have to do with oxidative injury? And what does the goddess Athena have to do with plasma microclots in peripheral smears?"

"Life *is* a miracle," he replied, his voice suddenly dropping to a whisper. "Creativity is a miracle. Advances in science are miracles and so are innovations in art. Newton, Einstein and Picasso understood that. And so did the ancient Greeks. You can understand that too, but first you have to learn something simple."

"What's that?"

"All knowledge is revealed. That's the universal and enduring truth. The laws of gravity were revealed to Isaac Newton. He neither saw nor felt gravity—no one can, for gravity is neither visible nor palpable. When relativity was revealed to Albert Einstein, he could touch neither time nor space—no one can. Sir Joseph John Thompson didn't invent the electron. He couldn't have seen the electron then."

"Hold it, Choua!" I said, annoyed. "I can't keep up with your wandering mind—or, should I say, with the shifting minds of the visiting ants? Come down to earth. Are the ants saying that learning anatomy, physiology and pathology isn't necessary in medicine?"

"On the contrary, learning the old knowledge paves the way for the revealed new knowledge," Choua replied, then added, "You physicians should learn from physicists, chemists and biologists. They have a better sense of the forever receding *absolute* truth. There is an assemblage of verifiable facts of anatomy, physiology, and pathology, and knowledge of them may be profitably employed in the care of the sick. But those basic sciences can't deliver to you the absolute truth about healing. The mystery, mystique and the miracle of healing extend far beyond the stark bits of knowledge in your medical texts. The sick know that intuitively. And so did you and your classmates when you went to medical school."

"What happened then?" I asked, puzzled.

"Your minds were sanitized by the gurus of the double-blinded and crossed-over drug studies."

"You have a one-track mind, Choua. You can't help being yourself, can you?" I rebuked him.

"You were indoctrinated to dismiss miracles because they might undermine your clinical authority."

"That's absurd," I countered. "You know I don't dismiss miracles. But there have to be some rigid standards in clinical medicine, some hard scientific criteria to see what works and what doesn't. The questions we face in clinical medicine are real, and so must the answers be."

"You don't get it, Mr. Pathologist, do you?" Choua frowned.

"Now what, Mr. Know-It-All?" I asked, nearly screaming in frustration.

"The mind can think only about what it knows. Just because one can see a question define itself, one isn't entitled to its answer." His face suddenly softened. "To know the miracle, you have to get past the mind." Choua smiled mysteriously, then slowly walked out of the room.

There are only two possibilities. First, that nothing is a miracle. Second, that everything is a miracle. I believe in the latter.

Albert Einstein,

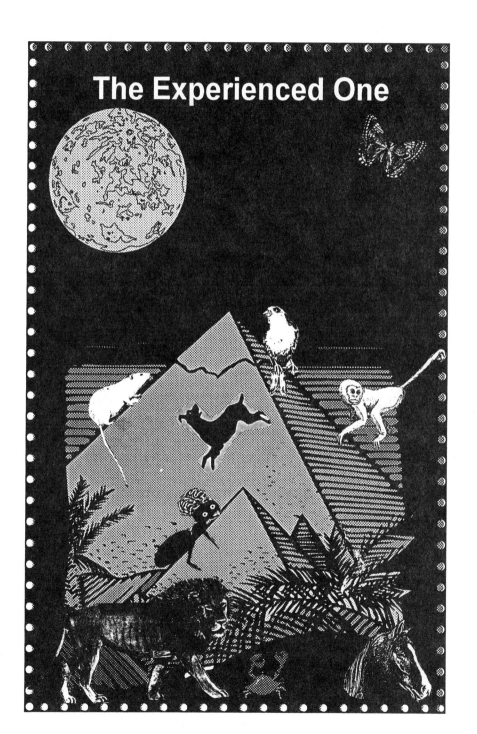

The Experienced One

I finished the preceding chapter entitled The Thinking Ants during my *Umrah* visit, a type of pilgrimage, in December 1996. While in Mekkah, Talat and I bought several books about the ancient and modern histories of Arabia and the Muslim holy cities of Mekkah *Mukkarama* and Medina *Munawwara*. While browsing in the bookstore, I thumbed through a book written by an American woman who had lived with Bedouins. Regrettably, I recall neither the name of the author nor her book. In the book I found the following story.

A Yemeni youth, who as a nine-year-old boy had learned to fend for himself and make a living doing errands, worked as a servant for a sick woman. She often asked him to go to the various physicians in town and bring them to her home for house calls, and very often she sent him to the *souk* to fetch medicine. Nothing seemed to work, and the woman remained sick and continued to suffer pain. One day he saw her in distress, thought about her afflictions and said to her,

"Why don't you consult the experienced one?"
"You know I have tried all the physicians in town. None of them could help me. Is there anyone left? Tell me about him and I'll try my luck with him," she replied.
"I mean the *Experienced One*," the youth went on.
"Who?" she asked, puzzled.
"*The Experienced One!*" The youth repeated. "The one who healed the sick long before there were any doctors or their drugs."

The more clinical work I do in integrative medicine, the more aware I become of what that Yemeni youth understood. *The Experienced One has more experience than I.*

What does the Experienced One whisper in the ears of this

inexperienced one? "You're a beginner. Marvel at the mystery of healing. Each time you see a patient, know that your knowledge is incomplete. Don't pride yourself on figuring out the answers—how can you do that when you cannot even ask the right questions? Recognize that you can think only about what you know."

"Science is purity of observation," the Experienced One adds. "But human observation is not infallible. Newton claimed that the armor of his science had no holes. Einstein looked for chinks in that armor and found some. At high speeds and strong gravities, Newtonian physics doesn't hold. Others are trying to find holes in Einstein's notions, and some will succeed."

"You have been wrong before," the Experienced One continues to whisper to the inexperienced one, "and you'll be wrong again. What is required of you is not healing, only an earnest effort to use whatever has been revealed to you. There is the *one* and only healer, and He isn't subordinate to your notions of healers and healing, nor to your schedule. You may facilitate healing—only by as much science and healing art as He bestows upon you. Knowing that, proceed with your work with the sick. Be humble when your therapies seem to work, because the same therapies do not work for some others. Your ability to care for the sick is a gift from Him. Be prepared to surrender it."

What is spirituality? No one can show anyone what is the spiritual, no one can make anyone else spiritual...There is, however, something about the spiritual that everyone can see and know—the visible reflection of the spiritual in the lives of those who go and return, not seeing anything, not hearing anything, not imagining anything, not knowing anything.

The Canary and Chronic Fatigue

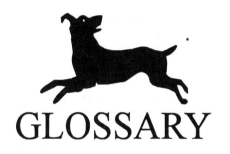

GLOSSARY

ADD:
>   Attention deficit disorder

AIDS:
>   **Acquired immune deficiency syndrome** generally believed to be
>   caused by HIV.

Abscess:
>   An inflammatory lesion which accumulates a pocket of pus.

Acid:
>   A substance that can react with alkalis to form salts, and can ionize to
>   give hydrogen ions. It turns litmus paper red.

Adaptation response (general):
>   A set of biochemical changes that is believed to prepare an organism to
>   cope with stress or a demand for change.

Adrenal glands:
>   A pair of glands weighing about one-half ounces and situated above the
>   kidneys. These glands produce adrenaline and steroid hormones. It is
>   commonly—and, in my view, inaccurately—believed to be the primary
>   body organ involved in the stress response.

Adrenaline rushes:
>   Blasts of adrenaline produced in sudden shock states that quicken the
>   heart rate, tighten the muscles and cause anxiety.

Adrenaline:
>   A hormone produced by the adrenal glands which plays many roles in
>   human biology, and is believed to cause the stress response.

Adrenaline roller coasters:
>   Repeated adrenaline rushes that follow each other, creating sharp peaks
>   and deep troughs of adrenaline levels in the blood and tissues.

Adrenergic hypervigilence:
>   A state of overproduction of adrenaline hormone and related hormones
>   that keeps various energy pathways revved up and causes molecular
>   burn-out.

Aging-oxidant molecules:
>   A family of oxidant molecules that cause death and decay in cells and
>   tissues. See oxidation.

Alkali:
>   A substance that can react awith acids to form salts, and can ionise to
>   produce hydroxyl radicals. It turns litmus paper blue.

All-in-the-head syndrome:
>   A derisive term used by many doctors to dismiss patients with chronic

complaints as malingerers—such symptoms are believed to be false and imaginary. See shirker's syndrome.

Amino acids:

Building blocks for proteins, amino acids are simple nitrogen-containing molecules.

Amitriptyline:

A tricyclic antidepressant drug. Brand name: Elavil.

Angina:

A painful condition of the heart which causes chest pain that often radiates to the left arm, left side of the face and/or neck. It is caused by inadequate blood supply to the heart due to spasm of coronary arteries or blockage caused by plaque.

Angioplasty:

A procedure by which an attempt is made to increase the blood supply to the heart by squeezing plaque in coronary arteries resulting in widening. Not recommended. Though theoretically a valid approach, it rarely works in real life because it does not address the underlying problems that cause heart disease.

Antihistamines:

A class of drugs that controls the symptoms of allergic reactions by blocking the action of histamine, a substance that is released from mast cells and, in turn, causes the release of many inflammation mediators.

Antibodies:

Proteins molecules produced in the body by the immune system to fight off microbial infections or deal with foreign materials. Antibodies are quite specific for the molecules against which they are directed.

Antioxidants:

Molecules that prevent oxidation (loss of electrons) of other substances. Antioxidants of interest in human metabolism include vitamins such as vitamins A, C and E as well as minerals such as selenium.

Antioxidant defenses:

Host defenses against oxidative molecular injury. See oxidation.

Anxiety state:

An abnormal state of undue anxiety about real or imagined adverse events. In severe forms, anxiety causes loss of appetite, difficulty with sleep, jitters, indigestion, heart palpitations and missed heart beats.

Arrhythmia:

Irregular heartbeat. Sometimes the individual can sense the irregular rhythm of the heart as skipped beats.

Arteriosclerosis:

Commonly called hardening of the arteries, arteriosclerosis is a disease process characterized by plaque formation on the inside walls of arteries. It leads to heart attacks, strokes and leg cramps while walking due to insufficient blood supply.

Ativan:

A commonly prescribed antianxiety drug. Generic name: lorazepam.

Attention deficit disorder:

A disorder of children as well as adults characterized by inattentiveness, impulsivity and inability to perform ordinary chores at home and at work. See hyperactivity syndrome.

Autism:

A disorder characterized by severe inability of the subject to react to ordinary stimulations and to communicate with family members and friends. The resulting isolation, unless averted, causes serious developmental problems.

Autoimmune disorders:

An individual's immunity turned against himself. A class of disorders in which an injured immune system produces antibodies directed against the body's own molecules, cells and organs. These autoantibodies may cause widespread tissue damage. See lupus, multiple sclerosis and hyperthyroidism.

Autonomic nervous system:

A part of the nervous system that is believed to be outside voluntary control, for example, nerve cells and nerve fibers that regulate normal heart rhythm and rate.

Autoregulation:

A process by which a person enters a healing energy state.

Azulfidine:

A drug used to suppress symptoms caused by various types of colitis such as ulcerative colitis, Crohn's colitis and others.

Biology:

A branch of science that deals with the structures and functions of living plants and animals.

Bite of the gray dog:

An autoregulation expression that refers to adverse effects—such as muscle spasm, tension, anxiety, abdominal cramps and others—that some people experience during the initial phases of meditation and spiritual work. These negative effects of autoregulation are usually short-lived.

Blood ecosystem:

A diverse, dynamic and delicate biochemical ecosystem of blood components circulating in blood vessels that actively interfaces with the bowel, liver, brain and other ecosystems. This concept contrasts with the traditional view that sterile blood circulates in a closed system of arteries and veins. The circulating blood is an open ecosystem in the sense that there is an ongoing free entry into it of bacteria, viruses and parasites from the bowel and other ecosystems of the body.

Bowel ecosystem:

A delicate, diverse and dynamic ecosystem composed of chemical (food elements and digestive-absorptive enzymes) and biologic elements (bacteria, viruses and parasites).

Bulbectomy:

An operation in which the olfactory bulb essential for the sense of smell is removed.

Cancer:

A malignant tumor that spreads and invades distant body organs. A growth produced by uncontrolled multiplication of cells.

Candida:

A single-celled fungus (yeast) normally found in the colon of almost all individuals. Furthermore, it is found in the blood stream of most persons with suppressed immune systems.

Capillary:

A minute blood vessel that represents the narrowest part of the vascular tree.

Cellular ecosystems:

The internal environment of cells and intracellular organelles that sense—and respond to—changes in the tissue fluid that bathes cells.

Cellulitis:

A type of inflammation which spreads rapidly within soft tissues, causing pain, swelling and redness—at times extending into the surrounding tissues as red streaks.

Chelation:

A process by which metals are eliminated from the body by binding them to substances with a special affinity for such metals. When used to reverse coronary artery disease, chelation employs EDTA as the chelating agent for calcium deposits in the plaque lining the arteries.

Chemotherapy:

Treatment with drugs used to control cancer. In general these drugs are highly toxic and seriously injure the immune system while incompletely killing cancer cells.

Cholesterol:

A waxy, fatty substance in the blood that is incorrectly considered to be the cause of heart disease, stroke and instances of common heart attacks.

Cholinergic:

A part of the autonomic nervous system that provides a counterbalance to adrenergic nerve receptors and messenger molecules such as adrenaline. See adrenaline.

Chronic fatigue syndrome:

A chronic state of undue tiredness that lasts for more than six months and results in more than a fifty percent reduction in physical activity. It is associated with immune dysfunctions; dysfunctions of the thyroid, adrenal and pancreas glands; and disorders of mood, memory and mentation.

Colitis:

Inflammation of colon which causes pain, abdominal bloating and cramps. Sometimes bleeding can occur.

Consciousness:

Traditionally defined as a state or condition of being critically aware of one's own identity and condition. In the context of autoregulation, it refers to an energetic awareness of one relationship with the larger *presence* around him.

Copernicus, Nicholaus (1473-1543)

A Polish mathematician and astronomer who discovered that the earth revolves around the sun, rather than the sun revolving around the earth as was believed by the ancient Egyptian Ptolemaic astronomers.

Coronary arteries:

Arteries that supply blood to the heart muscle.

Coronary artery disease:

A disease state created by inadequate blood supply to the heart caused by blockage of the coronary arteries by plaque formation.

Cortical:

In autoregulation terminology, cortical indicates a thinking state in which the mind counts, calculates, computes, competes, censors and cautions. The cortical mind creates images of suffering and disease. It is a competitive mode in which one yearns for control, further compounding the problem. In contrast, limbic in autoregulation terminology cares and comforts. It creates images of relief and health, and so mitigates suffering. In the limbic mode, human energy pathways are in a steady state and facilitate the healing response.

Cortical monkey:

In autoregulation terminology, it refers to a mind fixated on itself—cycling past misery unendingly and, when that is not enough, precycling feared, future misery.

Cortical overdrive:

In autoregulation terminology, it refers to relentless—and futile—worrying about things that do not happen.

Cylert:

A drug used for attention deficit and related learning disorders.

Cytomegalovirus:

A common virus that causes fever and may involve any body organ, especially when the immune system of the individual is compromised by antibiotic abuse, chemotherapy, radiotherapy and environmental toxins.

Decerebrate:

An animal in which a significant part or whole of the brain has been removed.

Dexedrine:

A drug (dextroamphetamine sulfate) that stimulates the nervous system and is often used for attention deficit disorder and related conditions.

DHEA:

Dehydroepiandrosterone, a "mother" hormone produced in the adrenal glands that orchestrates the production of estrogens, progesterones and testosterone in the body. It is also considered to be an anti-aging hormone.

Diagnostic labels:

The diagnostic terms that are employed in drug medicine to justify the use of symptom-suppressing drugs but reveal nothing about the cause of the illness. For instance, irritable bowel syndrome, chronic headache and restless leg syndrome.

Directed Pulses:

A term used in autoregulation to indicate enhancement and perception of ordinary arterial pulses in different parts of the body.

Distress:

A state of harmful stress, contrasted to eustress, which is believed to be a helpful state of stress.

Diuretics:

A class of drugs used to treat excessive accumulation of fluids in tissues. These drugs promote loss of fluids via the urine.

Dynamics:

The study of relationships between motion and the forces affecting the motion of physical systems.

Dysautonomia:

A disorder of autonomic nervous system that often causes disturbances in heart rate, blood pressure, sweating and control of urination.

Dysfunction:

Malfunction in the cells, tissues and organs.

Dysregulation:

Abnormalities in the regulation of various molecular functions in the body. For instance, ingestion or assimilation of external synthetic chemicals with estrogen-like activities interfere with normal hormonal functions in women and cause such disorders as endometriosis.

EDTA:

Ethylenediaminetetraacetic acid, a substance used in chelation therapy to eliminate toxic heavy metals in cases of metal poisoning, to remove calcium and reverse coronary heart disease.

Ecotoxins:

Toxic substances in the environment, including man-made synthetic molecules as well as some naturally produced toxins.

Ecology:

Study of relationships between living beings and their environment. In this volume, it is used to focus on inter-relationships between the various molecular, cellular and tissue systems of the human body.

Einstein, Albert (1879-1955):

A German-born U.S. physicist who showed that the mass of a body is a measure of its energy content. His theory of general and special relativity revolutionized our thinking about time and space.

Elavil:

A brand name for a tricyclic antidepressant drug called amitriptyline. Other brand-name drugs that contain amitriptyline include Endep, Etrafon, Limbitrol and Triavil.

Electrodemal conductance:
> An energy field created when two electrodes are attached to the skin of two different parts of the body. A method of testing for food incompatibilities is based on this phenomenon.

Electromagnetism:
> The study of electricity and magnetism. Also magnetism arising from an accelerating charge.

EM medicine (energetic-molecular medicine):
> A type of medical practice in which therapies are based on energetic-molecular events that occur *before* cells and tissues are damaged and disease develops, rather than on how tissues look under a microscope *after* they have been damaged.

EM traffic:
> Energetic-molecular events that take place at the cell and plasma membranes in health and disease, and represent the essential energy dynamics of living beings.

Endothelins:
> Substances produced in the blood vessel wall and other parts of the body that serve a large number of functions, such as the control of blood flow within arteries and the regulation of many hormonal functions.

Energy Responses:
> In autoregulation terminology, it refers to subtle energy that is perceived during meditation. In some areas as in simple hand warming, energy responses can be readily documented with suitable electronic equipment. In other areas, technology to measure such responses is not yet available.

Enzyme:
> Catalysts that facilitate biochemical reactions in the body. Enzymes are delicate proteins that are highly vulnerable to oxidant stress.

Epstein-Barr virus (EBV):
> A common virus that causes infectious mononucleosis (kissing disease), and was at one time thought to be the cause of chronic fatigue syndrome.

Estrogens:
> A class of female hormones essential for normal fetal development, and for maintenance of menstruation and other female reproductive functions. Opposed by progesterones.

ETS:
  See endothelins.

Eustress:
  Eustress is considered a type of stress with healthful effects.

Fatigue:
  Undue tiredness. Also see chronic fatigue syndrome.

Fourth-of-July Chemistry:
  A state of chemistry in which electrons are fired excessively and randomly in various tissues, causing widespread damage to cellular enzymes, membrane receptors, membrane channels, enzymes, hormones and neurotransmitters.

Gallileo Galilei (1564-1642):
  Italian mathematician and astronomer who discovered four satellites of Jupiter and the nature of lunar illumination. His support of Copernicus's assertion that the earth revolves around the sun led to his persecution by the Inquisition (1633).

Geomagnetism:
  The magnetism of the earth.

Glucaric acid:
  A substance that indicates increased detoxification activity by the liver enzymes. Increased urinary amounts are found in chronic fatigue states, chemical sensitivity and other states.

Glucose:
  A simple six-carbon sugar molecule that is utilized in the tissues for energy production. In the brain, glucose is almost exclusively utilized for all neurologic functions.

Glucose roller coasters:
  A term I use for rapid changes in the blood sugar level creating high peaks and deep valleys. Synonymous with rapid hyperglycemic-hypoglycemic shifts.

Growth hormone:
  A pituitary hormone that promotes growth during childhood and prevents premature aging.

HDL cholesterol:
  High-density lipoprotein, the "good" cholesterol that is supposed to prevent coronary heart disease. The higher the blood level, the lower the presumed risk of heart disease. I say presumed because this is an overly simplistic view.)

Herpesvirus:

A family of viruses that causes common fever blisters in the mouth as well as genital lesions.

High-energy molecule:

A molecule that contains chemical energy bonds that may be broken to release the energy contained in them. For example, glycogen is a high-energy molecule that contains many energy bonds. When it is broken down into smaller sugar molecules, energy is released for muscular activities or other energy functions in the body.

HIV:

HIV (human immunodeficiency virus) causes AIDS (acquired immunodeficiency syndrome).

HMO:

Health maintenance organizations, in essence, are insurance companies that specialize in reducing costs by controlling the spending of doctors.

Hormone:

A substance in the body that is produced by glands called endocrine glands. In the past deemed as a molecule that is produced in one organ and exerts its effects on another. Now some hormones are recognized as produced primarily for local effects, i.e., nitric oxide produced in endothelial cells lining blood vessels.

Hyperactivity syndrome:

A syndrome usually diagnosed in children whereby a child is restless, impulsive and unable to perform common chores at home or at school.

Hyperadrenergic state:

A state in which excessive release of adrenaline and related stress molecules causes restlessness, anxiety, insomnia, heart palpitations and stress.

Hypochondria:

Neurotic conviction of the existence of an imaginary illness. Derived from hypochondrium—a region of abdomen located below the cartilage of the breast bone—thought to be the seat of melancholy in the past.

Hyperglycemia:

Opposite of hypoglycemia. A state of raised blood sugar levels. Persistent hyperglycemia is the essential feature of diabetes.

Hyperthyroidism:

An autoimmune disorder characterized by overactivity of the thyroid gland that causes undue sensitivity to high temperatures, speeded-up metabolism, sweating, weight loss and heart palpitations. See autoimmune disorders.

Hypoglycemia:

Opposite of hyperglycemia. A state of low blood sugar—usually lower than 50 mg/Dl—associated with symptoms of weakness, jitters, anxiety, heart palpitations, nausea and sweating.

Hypothyroidism:

Opposite of hyperthyroidism. An autoimmune disorder characterized by underactivity of the thyroid gland that causes undue sensitivity to cold temperatures, fatigue, dry skin, weight gain, hair loss and sluggish metabolism.

Hysteria:

A type of neurosis characterized by vulnerability to suggestion, amnesia, emotional instability and related mental disturbances.

ICU:

Intensive care units in a hospital.

Immune system:

The Body's system of defense against microbes and foreign substances. Specifically it involves the body's production of antibodies to destroy microbes or neutralize foreign substances.

Immunology:

A discipline in medicine that deals with health and disease of the defense systems of living beings called the immune system.

Infarction:

Death of tissue due to the sudden interruption of its blood supply. Example: myocardial infarction causes heart attack.

Insulin:

A *storage* hormone produced in the pancreas that regulates blood sugar levels by promoting storage of glucose in tissues as fat. It also facilitates the entry and utilization of sugar in cells.

Insulin roller coasters:

Sharp peaks in blood insulin levels followed by precipitous drops, which represent the dysregulation of insulin production in the pancreas.

Ischemia:

A condition of diminished blood supply to tissues. Examples: ischemia of the heart muscle, which may cause heart attacks, and of the brain, which may lead to stroke.

Integrative medicine:

A medicine that integrates empirical knowledge of healing nutrients and herbs as well as energy methods with the science and technology of modern medicine. It prescribes what is safe and effective regardless of what disciplines the particular therapy may come from.

Jung, Carl Gustave:
Eminent swiss psychiatrist, an early friend of Freud, who later forcefully disagreed with many aspects of Freudian psychology.

Klonopin:
A drug used to improve the function of the brain neurotransmitter, GABA, and to promote sleep and control anxiety.

Language of silence:
In autoregulation terminology, it is an intuitive-visceral stillness that enlightens without any analytical activity: equivalent to a profound meditative state in other disciplines of meditation.

LDL cholesterol:
Low-density lipoprotein that is often considered "bad" cholesterol. A raised blood level of LDL is considered a risk factor for heart disease.

Leaky cell membrane syndrome:
A term used by the author for health disorders that can be traced to consequences of oxidative damage to cell membranes which increases cell membrane permeability and leads to hemorrhage out of the cell what belongs inside and flooding of cell innards by elements that do not belong to the cell. For example, functional deficiency of magnesium and potassium and functional excess of calcium in chemical sensitivity and mold allergy reactions—clinical situations in which supplemental magnesium and potassium and calcium channel blockers are effective.

Life span:
The length of one's whole life. For humankind, it has been estimated to be between 100 and 110 years.

Life span enzymes:
Enzymes that promote health and allow a living being to achieve his or her expected life span. Also see enzyme.

Limbic:
Limbic indicates a calm, comforting, noncompetitive healing energy state. The term autoregulation refers to a nonthinking, noncompetitive, nongoal-oriented, steady healing energy state. The limbic state "cares and comforts," and "creates" images of health and healing that mitigate suffering. The cortical state, by contrast, indicates a thinking state in which the mind counts, calculates, computes, competes, censors and

cautions. It creates images of suffering and disease. It is a competitive mode in which one yearns for control, further compounding the problem.

Limbic breathing:

In autoregulation terminology, a type of breathing that profoundly affects the energy state of an individual. Limbic breathing is an enhanced energy state in which the breathing-out phase of respiration is prolonged in a slow, sustained fashion following a brief effortless breathing-in period. Very effective for reducing stress, slowing quickened heart rates, normalizing high blood pressure, and managing other chronic disorders.

Limbic calmness:

In autoregulation terminology, it refers to peace and tranquillity that comes with meditative surrendering to the *presence* that permeates and surrounds each of us at all times.

Limbic exercise:

A type of nongoal oriented, noncompetitive exercise in which slow, sustained physical exercise is combined with meditation.

Limbic language of silence:

In autoregulation terminology, this expression refers to reaching higher energy states with periods of silence and meditation.

Limbic silence:

In autoregulation terminology, it refers to a deep state of visceral tranquillity in which there is no awareness of ordinary stress-inducing perceptions.

Limbic-Spiritual

In autoregulation language, a term for a non-thinking, non-analytical energy healing state to which one surrenders in silence to the larger *presence* that surrounds and permeates one's being.

Limbic-visceral:

In autoregulation terminology, a non-thinking energy state—but not quite as spiritual as the limbic-spiritual.

Low-energy molecule:

A molecule with few energy bonds or electrons available for transfer to other molecules. See high-energy molecule for further explanation.

Lupus:

An autoimmune disorder in which a confused immune system turns on the body's own tissues and produces destructive antibodies that damage

---

various body organs. Full medical name: systemic lupus erythematosus.

Malignant:

A term used for cancer, such as a malignant tumor.

Mantra:

A word or a short phrase that is repeated often in one's mind to induce a contemplative state. In Hinduism, mantras are used in prayers and incantations, and are believed to be sacred words that embody the divinity invoked.

MAO:

Monoamine oxidase (MAO) inhibitors are a class of antidepressant drugs.

MRI:

A type of exquisitely sensitive scan that utilizes magnetic energy for creating diagnostic images.

Melatonin:

A hormone produced in the pineal gland that promotes natural sleep during night hours. It also helps people and animals adjust to various seasons.

Mercapturic acid:

A substance that indicates increased demand for detoxification in the liver. Increased levels in the urine are seen in chronic fatigue syndrome, chemical sensitivity and many other conditions.

Metabolism:

The complex of biochemical and physical processes involved in the maintenance of life. Metabolism comprises reactions necessary for breakdown of food substances for release of chemical bond energy (catabolism) as well as those for synthesis of structural and functional molecules for cellular and tissue build-up (anabolism).

Metabolic Roller coasters:

This term is used in this volume for abrupt changes in the blood and tissue levels of sugar, insulin, adrenaline, cholinergic hormones and neurotransmitters. Sharp rises and sudden drops in the levels of such molecules cause a host of symptoms such as anxiety, the jitters, nausea, weakness, sweating and heart palpitations.

Metaphysical:

Based on abstract or speculative situations. Sometimes considered supernatural.

Microclot:

A microscopic clot composed of coagulated (curdled) blood plasma with or without blood cells entrapped within it.

Microplaque:

A microscopic plaque circulating in the blood stream composed of clotted blood plasma with entrapped blood platelets, dead and dying blood cells and microbes including yeast. Microplaques clog blood capillaries in various body organs and cause all patterns of tissue injury and symptomatology.

Mind-body-spirit:

A spurious concept of using the thinking mind to force healing on injured tissues.

Miracle:

A happening that is considered beyond the laws of nature. An act of God. In common language, an exceptionally fortunate event.

Mitral valve prolapse:

A condition in which a chronically overdriven heart muscle stresses the mitral valve. The mitral valve leaflets bulge (prolapse), become floppy, and fail to prevent the backflow of blood from the left lower chamber of the heart to the left upper chamber. Except when it is associated with a mitral valve damaged by rheumatic fever or other conditions, it is *not* a specific heart defect. The proper holistic approach is to address all the elements that overdrive the heart of each individual patient.

Molecules:

A group of atoms with defined atomic arrangement within its structure.

Morphology:

A scientific discipline that deals with the structure and appearance of living beings as well as nonliving entities.

Multiple sclerosis:

An autoimmune disorder that damages the insulation material in nerve fibers called myelin sheaths.

Murmur:

An abnormal heart sound produced by turbulence in the flow of blood within the heart. It may be caused when the heart is overdriven, when one of the heart valves does not open fully (stenosis), or when it does not close fully (regurgitation).

Myocardial infarction:

Death of the heart muscle; heart attack, in common terminology.

N²D² medicine:

A type of medicine in which a practitioner's work begins with a search for the name of a disease and ends with the selection of a name of a drug. In N²D² medicine, no consideration is given to the ecologic and nutritional factors in the cause of disease. This type of medicine is expressed as follows:

N²D² medicine=
Name of a disease X Name of a drug

In N²D² medicine, a doctor begins care of a patient with a disease name and ends with a drug name.

Natural selection:

According to Darwin's theory, natural selection is a phenomenon that results in the survival of the fittest individuals and species. Seen in light of modern genetics, natural selection refers to gene mutations that favor survival of the species and so preserve and prolong the survival of the new (genetically altered) species. Mutations that adversely affect the survival result in extinction (being selected out) of that species.

Neuron:

A nerve cell present in the brain and nerve ganglia of many body organs.

Neurotransmitters:

Molecules that facilitate communications between nerve cells.

Newton, Isaac (1642-1727)

English mathematician and physicist who described the laws of gravity and motion, and devised calculus independent of Leibnitz.

Nitric oxide:

1) A simple but essential molecule composed of one atom each of nitrogen and oxygen. In human tissues, it regulates the caliber of small blood vessels and so regulates blood pressure within normal limits. It also functions as a hormone in many different organs of the body.

2) A colorless gas composed of one molecule of oxygen and one of nitrogen. It is an important messenger molecule that is produced in the cells lining the blood vessels, brain, immune cells and many other organs. Among its many metabolic roles is regulation of blood circulation.

Obsessive-compulsive disorder:
>A type of neurosis in which the sufferer feels compelled to think or do nonsensical things. If such a compulsion is resisted, the individual becomes dysfunctional.

Organ ecosystems:
>An ecologic community of biochemical and biologic elements together with its physical environment situated within a specific body organ. For instance, liver ecosystem, brain ecosystem etc.

Ovary:
>An organ in the female pelvis that produces ova (eggs) for conception and various female hormones.

OSHA:
>Occupational Safety and Health Administration.

Oxidation:
>Loss of electrons (tiny packets of energy) from an atom or a molecule. In common language, it may be seen as decay of high-energy molecules into low-energy molecules. Oxidation in nature is a spontaneous process—it requires no outside programming. Examples of oxidation in nature include spoiled fruit, rotten fish, rancid butter, decomposed grass, and denatured energy enzymes that cause chronic fatigue.

Oxidative coagulopathy:
>A term used by the author for a state of accelerated oxidative coagulation of plasma proteins resulting in formation of protein coagulum, microclots and micro-plaques in the circulating blood. In author's view, this is the true cause of coronary heart disease in addition to most other chronic degenerative disorders.

Oxidative fires:
>A term I use for accelerated oxidative molecular injury that literally cooks enzymes, hormones and other essential molecules in the blood and tissues.

Oxidative injury:
>Injury to molecules and tissues in which the mechanism of the injury involves the oxidation or decay of high-energy molecules into low-energy molecules.

Oxygen:
>A colorless, tasteless gas that makes up about 80 percent of the air and 85 percent of water, that is necessary for oxidation in nature.

Palpitations:
>A rapid heart rate that causes an uncomfortable perception of heartbeats

in the chest.

Pancreas:

A gland situated behind the stomach in the upper abdomen that produces insulin, glucagon and other hormones for regulation of carbohydrate metabolism, as wellas digestive enzymes in the small intestines.

Panic attacks:

Attacks of extreme anxiety caused by fear of things that do not happen; for example, a sudden sense of doom and fear of heart attack when such an attack has been ruled out repeatedly.

Pantothenic acid:

Vitamin B_5. It is a precursor of Co-enzyme A, and thus is an essential component of the detoxification system.

Pyridoxin:

Vitamin B_6

Pathology:

The study of disease processes and their clinical and laboratory manifestations.

Paxil:

An antidepressant drug.

ph:

Measure of acidity and alkalinity of a solution. Neutral solutions have a ph value of 7. Its value is calculated as the common logarithm of the reciprocal of the hydrogen ion concentration in moles per cubic decimeter of solution.

Phlebitis:

Inflammation of the vein wall accompanied by clotting of blood within the vein. Clinically, it is recognized as painful, tender linear thickening extending along the vein wall.

Phobia:

An irrational, often morbid, fear of things that may or may not take place.

Photosynthesis:

A process by which sun light strikes and agitates chlorophyll molecules thus producing minute electric currents, which, in turn, split water in plants into oxygen and hydrogen. Oxygen escapes into the atmosphere while hydrogen is combined with carbon dioxide to form sugar molecules. Thus is created the chemical bond energy of plants which begins the food chain on planet earth.

Physiology:
The branch of biology concerning the function of organisms.

Picasso, Pablo (1881-1973)
Spanish painter who is widely accepted as the prodigious master of 20th century art.

Pineal gland:
A gland located near the base of the brain that produces a hormone called melatonin to induce sleep as well as other hormones.

Plaque:
An area of swelling involving the inner lining of an artery caused by tissue injury and accumulation of oxidized and denatured fats, with or without surface ulceration or blood clot formation.

Platelets:
Irregularly shaped particles in circulating blood that contain essential blood clotting factors.

PMS:
Premenstrual syndrome consisting of irritability, cramps, headache, mood swings and water retention that often precedes the menstrual flow. PMS is caused by hormonal imbalance.

PPO:
Preferred provider organization. An organization of health care providers established for the purpose of standardizing provider fees.

Precycling feared future misery:
In autoregulation terminology, it is a neurotic compulsion to indulge in disturbing thoughts about the future.

Prilosec:
An antiulcer drug that works by inhibiting the proton pump involved in the production of stomach acid. Generic name: omeprazole.

Progesterone cream:
A progesterone cream derived from wild yam.

Progesterones:
A class of female hormones that provide a counterbalance to another class of female hormones called estrogens.

Prostate:
A gland in male mammals that secretes a fluid which becomes a part of semen. In men, it is the size of a walnut and is located at the neck of the urinary bladder. Both benign prostate enlargement and prostate cancer are quite common. In the author's view, the current pandemic of

prostate cancer in men is due to an excess of synthetic estrogens and xenoestrogens in the environment.

Protoplasm:

Thick fluid that is the soup of life in all living beings. It performs most of the basic life functions.

Prozac:

An antidepressant drug.

Psyche:

In Greek mythology, an exceedingly beautiful maiden loved by and later united with the Greek god, Eros. Later she became the personification of the soul.

Psychoneuroimmunology:

A branch of medical science that deals with links among aspects of the psyche, the brain and the immune system.

Psychosomatic:

A disease process that is assumed to be caused by disorders of the mind.

Pustule:

An inflammatory pimple that accumulates pus and usually appears as a lesion with white-gray center surrounded by swollen, red tissues.

Quran:

The holy book of Islam. It is the sacred text of revelations made by Allah to Prophet Muhammad. The holy book is often referred to as the Koran by nonmuslims.

RDA:

An abbreviation for the recommended daily allowance, RDA refers to amounts of nutrients considered sufficient to prevent a handful of nutrient deficiency diseases. RDA is the prevailing —and a pernicious—notion that holds that nutrients play no roles in the healing phenomena in injured tissues, and thus are of no value in the clinical management of ecologic, immune and nutritional disorders.

Reactive hypoglycemia:

Abnormally low level of blood sugar thought to be caused by anxiety and emotional disorders. True hypoglycemia, by contrast, is considered to be caused by a dysfunction of the pancreatic release of insulin. This distinction in my view is artificial and clinically irrelevant.

Receptors:

Molecules that provide "docking" sites for attachment to cell membranes for hormones and related substances. For example, receptors for estrogen and progesterone hormones.

Reduction:

In scientific chemistry terminology, the term reduction refers to the gain of electrons by molecules—the opposite of oxidation. When oxidation and reduction occur together, it is called a redox reaction.

Relaxation response:

A set of exercises designed to reduce stress and a set of biochemical changes associated with relaxation described by Harvard professor, Herbert Benson, M.D.

Resonance:

The quality of enhancement of response of a system to a periodic driving force when the driving frequency is equal to the frequency of the system. In autoregulation terminology, it is the energy response of molecules, cells and tissues to energy fields that surround them.

Ritalin:

A drug that stimulates the nervous system and is used for patients with attention deficit disorder.

Selye, Hans:

A noted stress expert credited with popularizing the fight-or-flight stress response.

Serengeti:

A large wildlife preserve in Kenya and Tanzania in East Africa.

Shirker's syndrome:

A derogatory term used to describe patients who complain of undue tiredness, and who are erroneously labeled by their physicians as malingerers.

Silence of stone:

In autoregulation terminology, it is a method of achieving an intuitive-visceral stillness by simply looking at a stone. No attempt is made to banish one's thoughts during this practice.

Somatic nervous system:

A part of the nervous system that is under voluntary control. Examples: use of legs for walking and of hands for holding.

Somatization:

Development of bodily dysfunction in response to emotional triggers.

Somatopsychic:

An adjective for organic medical conditions that secondarily affect the mind.

Spirituality:
> Dimensions of human existence that cannot be perceived by physical senses and are beyond the reach of human intellect. I consider spirituality to be the linkage with that larger presence that surrounds and permeates each of us at all times. In my view, it has nothing to do with clever thinking and is quite distinct from intellectual achievement.

Spontaneity of healing:
> A natural healing phenomenon that occurs without external aid. In essence, all healing is spontaneous.

Spontaneity of living:
> A philosophy of life that fosters heeding natural impulses of essential human goodness. In autoregulation terminology, it is living a life uncensored by the cortical monkey.

Spontaneity of oxidation:
> A natural phenomenon in which high-energy molecules spontaneously undergo decay and are turned into low-energy molecules.

Steroids:
> Also **known** generically as cortisone. These are a family of powerful hormones produced by the adrenal gland, ovaries, testes and some other body organs that perform a large variety of hormone functions in the body, including maintaining sexual functions.

Stress:
> Usually defined as a fight-or-flight response to demand for change. The term was coined by Walter Cannon and popularized by Hans Selye. In this book, stress is regarded as the essential process of decay and dying in living beings—the injury-healing-injury cycle of life.

Stress test (of the heart):
> A test for adequacy of the blood supply to the heart muscle. In this test, the heart is first stressed by exercise (treadmill or exercise cycle) and then its performance is evaluated with a cardiogram or a thallium scan.

Syndrome of just being sick:
> A term first coined and later abandoned by the noted stress expert, Hans Selye.

Taurine:
> A derivative of the amino acid cysteine, 2-aminoethane sulfonic. It is an important cell membrane stabilizer which is found in all cells. For this reason it is liberally used in clinical nutritional medicine. Taurine was so named because it was first isolated from ox bile (*taurus* in Latin

means bull.)

T$_3$:

A hormone produced by the thyroid gland to regulate metabolism and body temperature. It is formed by the breakdown of its parent (precursor) hormone called T$_4$.

T$_4$:

Thyroxine hormone produced by the thyroid gland to regulate metabolism and body temperature.

TPR:

An abbreviation for tumor potential normalization.

Thallium scans of the heart:

A type of heart scan that shows patterns of circulation in the heart muscle and is used for diagnosing coronary artery disease.

Thyroid gland:

A gland situated in the front of the neck that produces hormones to regulate metabolism. Underactivity of the gland is called hypothyroidism; overactivity is called hyperthyroidism.

Tourette's syndrome:

A syndrome characterized by involuntary muscular twitches, ticks, learning disabilities and uncontrollable use of foul language.

Trigger Points:

Chronically painful and tender areas located in sprained or partial torn ligament, tendons and muscles.

Triglycerides:

A type of fatty substance in the body which, when present in excessive amounts, is considered to be a risk factor for common heart attacks and strokes. In my view, this risk is grossly exaggerated by physicians who prefer to prescribe drugs rather than take a natural approach to the prevention of heart disease.

Tumor board:

A hospital board of physicians belonging to different specialties that meets to discuss diagnosis of tumors and plan treatment. Although an excellent concept in theory, the author has rarely seen it contribute significantly to any patient's actual care.

Valium:

An antianxiety drug. Generic name: diazepam.

Varicose:

Dilated and tortuous veins in which blood may stagnate and lead to phlebitis.

Vasodilatation:

Opening up of blood vessels—a process of relaxation of the muscle in the walls of arteries that results in improved blood circulation and oxygenation of tissues.

Vasospasm:

Spasm of the blood vessels.

Viruses:

A family of microbes that cannot be seen with ordinary microscopes and generally can thrive only within the host's cells. Examples: HIV, EBV, CMV and herpesviruses.

Visceral-Intuitive

In autoregulation terminology, it refers to an energy state in which enlightenment comes though non-analytical mediums. Also see Limbic-Visceral and Limbic-Spiritual.

Yeast:

Any of the single-celled fungi. In the opinion of the author, among the four groups of microbial invaders of the human body (viruses, bacterial, yeast and parasites), yeast pose the most significant threat to human health.

Zoloft:

An antidepressant chemically unrelated to tricyclic and tetracyclic antidepressants. Generic name: sertraline hydrochloride.

Humankind needs the language of silence today more than at any time during its history. We cannot "clever-think" our way out of all of our problems. The cortical monkey loves to recycle past misery. When that's not enough, it loves to precycle feared, future misery. We simply think too much. There are times we need the limbic language of silence.

The Goraa and Limbic Exercise

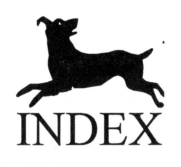

INDEX

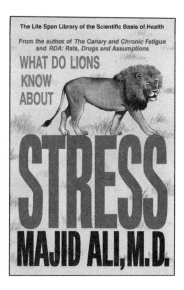

"The work of a master storyteller...a sort of Aesop of medicine...teaches highly effective methods for stress control."

Professor Alfred O. Fayemi
Mount Sinai School of Medicine, New York

"A wonderfully readable book about controlling stress...Ali's animals will teach you more about the hard science of stress than any other book on the subject."

Professor Francis Waickman
Northeastern Ohio University College of Medicine

What Do Lions Know About Stress
Majid Ali, M.D.
ISBN 1-879131-10-2
550 Pages

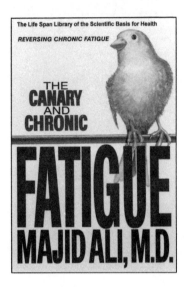

The definitive book on chronic fatigue!

"I am awestruck by the elegant simplicity of Dr. Ali's theory. With solid clinical outcome studies, he shows how non-drug therapies succeed in reviving injured energy enzymes where drugs fail. This book is a triumph of reason and common sense in medicine."

Ralph Miranda, M.D.
President, The American College for the Advancement in Medicine

"This 'textbook' of chronic fatigue simply must be read by everyone who sufferers from fatigue and everyone who cares for fatigue sufferers."

Kendall Gerdes, M.D.
President, The American Academy of Environmental Medicine

The Canary and Chronic Fatigue
Majid Ali, M.D.
ISBN 1-879131-04-8
580 pages

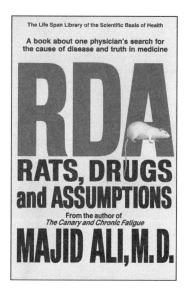

First time published heart scans of reversal of coronary artery disease with EDTA chelation.

"A courageous and brutally honest statement on the sad state of affairs of drug medicine in America."
Walter Ward, M.D.
Past President, American Academy of Otolaryngic Allergy

"Ali's documentation of reversal of advanced coronary artery disease is timely. Rats may save a lot of people from unnecessary coronary bypass surgery."
Alfred O. Fayemi, M.D.
Vice President, American Academy of Preventive Medicine

RDA: Rats, Drugs and Assumptions
Majid Ali, M.D.
ISBN 1-879131-07-2
670 pages

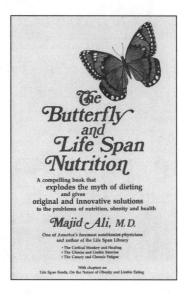

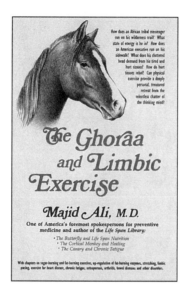

A wonderful book about the joys of fitness without the cortical burdens of goals.

"Clearly this book teaches us how to listen and tap into our inner self, letting it be the guide to life. Excellent book."
William J. Rea, M.D.
Author, *Chemical Sensitivity*

"At last a book that helps you discover the exhilaration of motion for motion's sake."
Robert C. Atkins, M.D.
Author, *Dr. Atkins' Health Revolution*

The Ghoraa and Limbic Exercise
Majid Ali, M.D.
ISBN 1-879131-02-1
335 pages

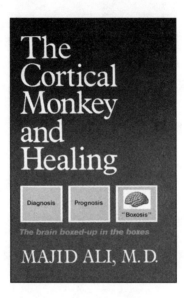

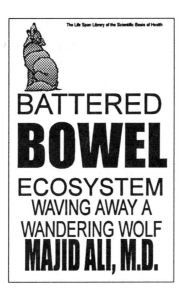

Coming Soon

Battered Bowel Ecosystem, Waving Away A Wandering Wolf
Majid Ali, M.D.

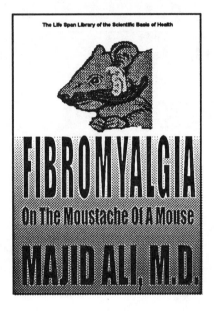

Coming Soon

Fibromyalgia:
On The Moustache Of A Mouse

Majid Ali, M.D.

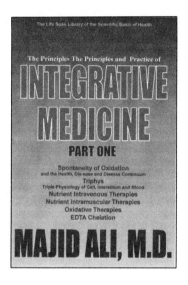

Intravenous and intramuscular formulas for specific autoimmune and chronic disorders.

Specifically written for the practicing health care professional.

The Principles and Practice
of Integrative Medicine
Majid Ali, M.D.

ISBN 1-879131-13-7

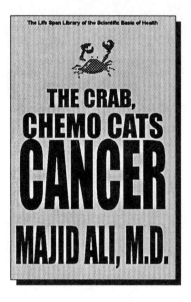

Coming Soon

The Crab, Chemo Cats and Cancer
Majid Ali, M.D.

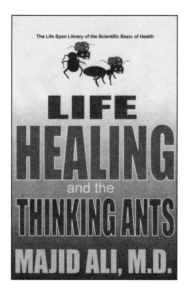

Coming Soon

Life, Healing and the Thinking Ants
Majid Ali, M.D.

A simple guide to life

ISBN 1-879131-09-9

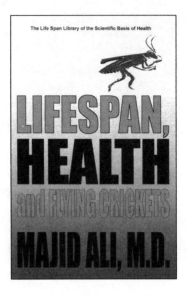

Coming Soon

Lifespan, Health
and Flying Crickets

A simple guide to health

ISBN 1-879131-12-9

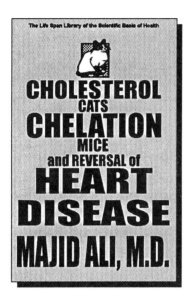

Coming Soon

Cholesterol Cats, Chelation Mice and Reversal of Heart Disease

Majid Ali, M.D.

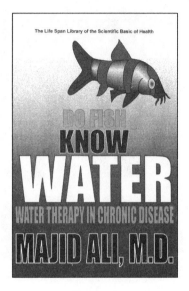

Coming Soon

Do Fish Know Water

Water therapy in chronic disease